Men on Sex

Men on Sex

Everything you ever wanted to ask...
THE *Esquire* REPORT

John Nicholson and
Fiona Thompson

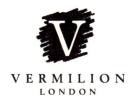

VERMILION
LONDON

Published in 1992 by Vermilion
an imprint of Ebury Press
Random House
20 Vauxhall Bridge Road
London SW1V 2SA

Copyright © John Nicholson and Fiona Thompson and
The National Magazine Company Limited 1992

John Nicholson and Fiona Thompson have asserted their right to be
identified as the author of this work in accordance with the
Copyright, Designs and Patents Act 1988.

All rights reserved. No part of the publication may be reproduced,
stored in a retrieval system, or transmitted in any form or by any
means, electronic, mechanical, photocopying, recording or otherwise,
without prior permission of the copyright owners.

Catalogue record for this book is available from the British Library.

ISBN 0 09177438 1

Typeset in Ehrhardt by SX Composing Ltd, Rayleigh, Essex
Printed in England by Mackays of Chatham Plc, Kent

Contents

FOREWORD BY ROSIE BOYCOTT	vii
INTRODUCTION	ix
1 Men and Women in the 90s	1
2 A Question of Priorities	12
3 First Bite at the Cherry	23
4 The Numbers Game	30
5 The Nitty Gritty	41
6 A Bit of What You Fancy	55
7 Sexual Types (or It Takes All Sorts)	67
8 Can Men Give Women What They Want?	94
9 Let's Talk About Sex	105
10 Dream Girls	116
11 Danger! Men at Play	123
12 Danger! Men at Work	140
13 And Then There Were Three	154
14 Down Your Way	166
INDEX	175

Foreword

When I became the editor of *Esquire* in January this year, one of the first projects I initiated was a MORI study into men's sexual attitudes in Britain.

As a founder of *Spare Rib* magazine, I have watched all the changes in women's lives and sexuality over the last two decades. These changes have been extensively documented. But what about men? Every change for women has meant a reciprocal change for men. We wanted to find out what these changes have added up to. Is the new man a reality or just an advertising concept? Is he still the same old man, wearing new clothes?

When I first talked to Dr John Nicholson, these were just some of the answers we were looking for. The results were illuminating and provide a unique insight into the sex lives of British men in the nineties.

Rosie Boycott
Editor, *Esquire*
1992

Introduction

Straightforward information on male sexuality is hard to come by. A few years ago, men could glean snippets from women's glossy magazines or try to sort the truth from the bravado of locker-room talk. Now, a new breed of men's magazines is widening the debate with straight-talking, hard-hitting facts. This book aims to provide the basis for further discussion at a time when so many areas of masculinity are chaotic, changing and challenged.

What do British men think about sex? How active are they in the sexual arena? What turns them on – in real life and in their fantasies? What happens to their sexual urges as they marry, have children and get older? What sexual variations tickle their fancy? And how much use do they make of sex aids, raunchy books or videos? Are there important differences in sexual practices between different parts of the country or different positions in the social pecking order?

What does your average middle-class man really think about women? Is he threatened by them, pleased to find himself working alongside them – or simply baffled by them? Does he know what turns women on, and if so, does he reckon he has what it takes?

To answer these and many other questions, we made contact with more than 800 British men at the end of 1991 and the beginning of 1992. Some completed a lengthy questionnaire, in a national survey conducted by the field force of MORI, others took part in small group discussions. In order to get a statistically reliable sample, we confined ourselves to one section of the population – the middle class – as defined in industry and advertising standards. Aged between 18 and 45, the sample formed a carefully selected, statistically valid sample of sexual behaviour and attitudes across England, Scotland and Wales. Findings of the national survey were further examined in small focus groups carried out in the South-East of England.

We also wanted to check our findings on some of the

subjects particularly relevant to men today. We found out what the sample thinks of changing roles in the workplace and the family, the number of partners a man has, and the effects of AIDS on sexual behaviour. But what does this mean for the man in the street? We chose four ordinary men as a 'first response group' to criticise, confirm or deny the evidence brought to light in the survey. You'll see their comments at the end of Chapters Four, Eleven, Twelve and Thirteen.

Men today are willing to talk about sex, and they do so sensibly, with insight and a surprising amount of humility. Almost 80 per cent of those who completed our questionnaire said they found the experience interesting; only 1 per cent were offended by it. In small groups, too, men are able to discuss intimate matters, whether the group leader is a man or a woman.

THE SAMPLE

Completed questionnaires of 786 men were subjected to comprehensive statistical analysis. All are between 18 and 45. Twenty-nine per cent are 18-24; 19 per cent 25-29; 17 per cent 30-34; 17 per cent 35-39; and 19 per cent between 40 and 45. The men involved come from 65 different points throughout England, Scotland and Wales (22 points in Scotland and the North of England, 16 points in the Midlands and Wales, 27 in the South). The major findings of the questionnaire were tested in small group discussions involving 35 people in six groups, held in the South-East of England.

Where percentages in tables or answers to questions do not add up to 100 per cent, this may be due to computer rounding, to the exclusion of certain categories such as 'don't know', or as a result of multiple response answers.

Two-thirds of the sample describe themselves as head of their households. Eighty-five per cent are in full-time employment; 7 per cent are students; only 3 per cent describe themselves as unemployed. Their average working week is 43.35 hours.

Ten per cent are not currently earning; 31 per cent earn up to £15,000; 21 per cent £15,000-£20,000; 15 per cent between £20,000 and £25,000; 9 per cent between £25,000 and £30,000; 6 per cent between £30,000 and £40,000; and 2 per cent are earning between £40,000 and £50,000. Four per cent of the sample are currently earning more than £50,000.

Thirty-one per cent have degrees; 71 per cent have at least 'O' levels; while only 6 per cent have no formal educational qualification whatsoever. More than 40 per cent had lived away from home by the time they were 18; 14 per cent were still living at home at the time of the survey.

The following 'cross-breaks' were applied across the questionnaire to pinpoint particular groups of men:

AGE: 18-24; 25-29; 30-34; 35-39; 40-45.

EDUCATION: *Basic* – Just 'O' levels/CSEs/GCSEs or no formal qualifications at all; *Middle* – 'A' level/OND/HND, but no higher; *Higher* – Degree/higher degree/other diploma.

INCOME: Up to £15k per year; £15-25k; over £25k.

EMPLOYMENT: *Higher* – Higher managerial/administrative/professional and head of household; *Middle* – Intermediate managerial/administrative or professional and head of household; *Lower* – Supervisor or clerical, junior managerial/administrative/professional, skilled manual, semi and unskilled manual, unemployed and head of household.

MARITAL STATUS: Married; cohabiting; separated/divorced/widowed; single.

FATHER: Father; non father.

LIVING WITH CHILDREN: Under four only; under nine only; any 10 or over; living together but no kids.

RELATIONSHIP: Regular; occasional; none; regular plus other relationship.

EXPERIENCE (sexual partners): One; two to four; five to nine; ten plus.

SEXUAL ACTIVITY: Four plus days a week; two to three days a week; one day a week; once or twice a month; less than once a month; never.

LOSS OF VIRGINITY: *Early* – Before 16; *Average* 16-19; *Late* – 20 plus.

FIRST-TIME ENJOYMENT: Great deal; fair amount; a little or not at all.

(N.B. Throughout, the 'separated' category includes separated and divorced men. It also includes the four widowed men in our sample.)

Bear in mind that some of the cross-breaks contain relatively small numbers. As a result, we cannot be sure that what is said by the individuals in such a group is representative of this section of men in society as a whole.

What does the survey tell us about the lifestyle of middle-class men in the UK today? Well, they reckon they're in pretty good shape physically; just one in five worry about being unfit, and only a third consider that they're even slightly overweight. Those who rarely have sex are particularly likely to say they're very fit! Whereas older men are the most likely to say they're overweight, men earning the least and those who rarely have sex tend to believe they're underweight.

Nearly six out of ten of our sample take exercise regularly; and they are surprisingly controlled in their use of the most popular psychopharmacological remedy – alcohol. The amount a man drinks varies very little through different age groups, but men in managerial positions and those earning more than £25k are considerably more likely to drink four times a week or more than others in the sample. Slightly more than a quarter of the men in our sample smoke cigarettes.

Forty-eight per cent of our sample are married, and the following table shows that among those aged 30 or more, the majority are married.

AGES OF MARRIED MEN	
18-24	7%
25-29	38%
30-34	64%
35-39	76%
40-45	82%

Ten per cent have live-in lovers, though men in their 40s are the least likely to be cohabiting with a partner outside marriage. Seven per cent of married or cohabiting men are unfaithful to their partners, and these men tend to be those who've had more than ten sexual partners. Infidelity is also linked to an early, enjoyable loss of virginity. The 3 per cent of the sample who are having a relationship with someone who is living with or married to someone else are particularly likely to be earning over £25k, to be separated, those who've had more than ten partners, and men who lost their virginity early and enjoyed it. Five per cent of the sample are divorced or separated, and three-quarters of this group have regular or occasional sexual partners. Thirty-six per cent of the sample are single, and this group includes four in five of men aged 18-24, two-thirds of unemployed men, and three-quarters of the men who have sex less than once a month. Five per cent of the sample are virgins.

Forty-three per cent are fathers (not necessarily living with their children), and this group includes a high proportion of men earning over £25k. Fifty-two per cent live in households which do not include children. Ninety-four per cent of the men describe themselves as exclusively heterosexual; 2 per cent are homosexual; 1 per cent are not interested in sex at all; and the remaining 3 per cent are bisexual. Ninety-nine per cent of married men say they're heterosexual; the rogue 1 per cent describe themselves as somewhat interested in men. Homosexuals make up 6 per cent of the cohabitors, 2 per cent of single men, and 6 per cent of the two-timers. Among those who've had more than ten sexual partners, there are more sexual ambiguities, as is shown below.

SEXUALITY ACCORDING TO EXPERIENCE

	'10 PLUS PARTNER' MEN	ONE-WOMAN MEN
Heterosexual	92%	98%
Bisexual	4%	1%
Homosexual	2%	–
Not interested	2%	1%

One man in five lost his virginity under the age of 16. Eighteen per cent have confined themselves to one sexual partner; 10 per cent have had more than 20; half have had between two and nine; 7 per cent are unable to make a reliable estimate! During the last year, more than two-thirds had remained faithful to a single partner.

Just over half the men in our sample consider themselves fairly highly sexed, and this category includes a high proportion of men earning over £25k and two-timers. The men most likely to say they're very highly sexed include unemployed people, those who've had more than ten partners, men who have sex at least four times a week, and those who lost their virginity before they were 16. The least highly-sexed group encompasses men without a relationship, those with very young children, men who never have sex and those who lost their virginity after the age of 19.

1.

Men and Women in the 90s

What's a man supposed to do? It's impossible to ignore the changes that have taken place in women's roles over the past 30 years. But where do men fit in? A man in his 20s today will have grown up taking these ideas on board. But for some older men, the social and sexual revolutions are harder to swallow, as they see women seeming to usurp their power base and doing things their mother (or wife) would never have done. To get a fix on men's attitudes now, we looked at men's and women's roles in the eyes of the young, the old, the rich, the poor, the married and the unattached.

We've seen a range of media stereotypes to define men. Firstly, there's the Male Chauvinist Pig who wants women in the home and in their place. Then we have the New Man – caring and sharing, with a baby in one hand and a tea towel in the other. Somewhere in the middle, there's the hybrid New Lad, who has time for both football and feminism. More recently, there has been the appearance of the 'Iron John' movement; this is for men who feel they need to reassert their right to be male, and could be the nearest thing yet to male liberation. Another issue to take into account is the current backlash against feminism, whereby men who feel women's demands have got out of hand are taking the offensive and staking out their masculine territory.

THE MALE ROLE

In this climate of change where some men feel the need to re-

MEN ON SEX

examine and redefine their roles, there is bound to be an effect on their attitudes towards women in a sexual and social context. So, as a first step towards analysing men's feelings about what constitutes a 'male' role, we asked them in which situations they feel most masculine. The following table shows their replies:

I FEEL MOST MASCULINE . . .	
During sport/physical exercise	45%
In bed	37%
At work	35%
Out socialising with my partner	25%
In a pub	23%
While driving	23%
Doing DIY/gardening	14%
At home	14%
With my children	10%
On holiday	9%
Other	5%

    Men in the group discussions agreed that team sports can be a powerfully 'masculine' experience. 'When you're doing something physical you do feel masculine,' according to a married 37 year old. 'You feel you're participating in a man's game, with other men. You feel like one of the lads, there is an air of masculinity about it. It's not a conscious thing – you feel good about yourself.' This was also the opinion of a married 32 year old in one of the groups: 'I used to play football and if you played well – if you scored or had a good pass – you had the adulation of your team mates. I remember I played at Villa Park and scored a goal, and the first person I looked for in the stand was my missus! I felt masculine then.'
    Professional footballer John Salako is better placed than most to expound on men testing their mettle in the field. 'Male bonding – what I call team spirit – is something that grows naturally in a sport like football. You've got to stick together.' He then adds, 'When I'm playing, I feel very confident. I get a buzz from the

sport, but it's more personal and professional satisfaction than some macho ego trip.'

Olympic gold medallist yachtsman Mike McIntyre makes some bolder claims for the power of men racing together: 'Sport is war without the violence. Comradeship happens naturally with a team of good men all working together for a goal. It's the same feeling you get in battle.'

But 'all-men-together' sports were felt to be just one way of expressing masculinity. In contrast with the rating given by the sample, most men in the groups said they could feel equally masculine in bed or with their children. As a married 33 year old pointed out: 'It depends what you mean by masculine. When I'm completely at ease with myself and I can be me, then I feel that's me. I'm masculine now – and you don't have to *feel* masculine, you just are what you are. And when I'm with the kids I'm like that. I can do what I like, I can laugh and joke with them because nobody's going to criticise me.'

The whole idea of 'masculinity' also came in for some ridicule from comments on the questionnaires, such as 'Never!', or this observation from a married man in his early 30s: 'It is not something that I often think about, and anyway, this depends on one's definition of "masculine".' And in one of the group discussions, a married 31 year old gained general approval when he asked, 'Don't you think "being masculine" is a phoney image?'

According to the sample, older men feel more manly in domestic situations – in bed, at home, doing DIY or gardening and with their children – whereas men in their late 20s score highest in sporting activities, socialising with their partner and being in a pub. They are also the most likely to say they feel masculine at work, which ties up with their fantasies as described in Chapter Ten. The more a man earns, the better he feels about his masculinity at work and with his children. However, the highest earners feel least good during sport and in pubs.

Young and single men, and particularly those who've had more than ten partners, are the most likely to conform to the boy racer stereotype. Men in the groups did think that driving could make them feel masculine, but noted that it had to be the right kind of car. Driving their wife's little runaround, for example, was unlikely to make their blood race! Power, speed and value were what mattered when it came to feeling masculine while driving: 'If you're sat in a Ferrari, you're masculine whether you're down the King's Road or whether you're on the motorway,' said a married 32 year old. According to a married 27 year old, the masculinity factor increases, 'if you've got a nice car and you're driving quick and you're showing off'. He continued, 'I'm fortunate enough to have a nice car. I don't mind admitting it's not bad for a guy of my age to be driving round in £15,000 worth of car.'

However, not everyone in the groups subscribed to the racing testosterone theory: 'To me, it's the Julie Walters "BCSD" syndrome, Big Car, Small Dick. All on the outside, not much on the inside,' was the acid comment of a married 33 year old.

Single men are particularly likely to say they feel masculine while driving and when on holiday. A third of them feel manly in the pub. By contrast, married men feel masculine at work, at home and with their children. An interesting statistic to emerge from the survey is that men who didn't enjoy losing their virginity are more likely to feel masculine during sport, whereas those who had a good first experience of sex are more likely to say they feel virile in bed.

The more often a man has sex, the more manly he feels in bed: half the men who have sex at least four times a week feel masculine in bed, compared with a tiny 9 per cent of men who never have sex. The men with the most sexual activity also feel more virile than most when they're out socialising with their partner. By contrast, men who've had the most partners feel more masculine than the rest in a pub. It's interesting that the highly sexually active link feelings of masculinity with their partner, while the most experienced opt for a place where they are likely to meet *more* partners!

MALE VERSUS FEMALE

'A lot of British men have this great arrogance,' according to fashion designer Paul Costelloe. 'They live in their own world, blind to changed attitudes about women. They've been brought up in a tradition of total male chauvinist piggery and they pretty much see women as mothers, nannies or tarts.' We asked about a range of issues from power to positive discrimination to discover where men in our sample stand.

WHO GETS THE BEST DEAL?

MEN	WOMEN	IT'S EQUAL	DON'T KNOW
68%	8%	16%	7%

Two-thirds of the sample say that men get the best deal in Britain today. When asked a supplementary question about the balance of power between the sexes, 56 per cent say it's too much in favour of men, 29 per cent think it's about right, 8 per cent don't know and just 6 per cent believe it's tipped too far in favour of women.

These questions inspired a few men to write comments at the end of their questionnaires. A separated 26 year old from the South East said: 'I feel there are certain areas where men get a better deal and others where women benefit. For instance, because men are caught in their masculine roles, then this often means men have very little room to develop their feminine side, i.e. expressing emotions, feelings etc., whereas women have plenty of room to develop these qualities. On the other hand, women have had a very raw deal living in a male-dominated society and so have difficulty climbing up the promotion ladder. There are lots of pros and cons.'

A 26 year old who lives with his partner in the North East feels that women have an advantage when it comes to learning about sex: 'I find it strange that women, particularly young females, have access to lots of information on sex and boys have far less.' There are other areas where women definitely have the upper hand, according to a single 22 year old from Scotland: 'Socially, women have by far been given too many rights concerning children – for example, custody, maintenance, power over access.'

Women on Top

The men among the *least* likely to feel they've got the best deal are those with basic education, men in lower forms of employment and the unemployed. These groups are also more likely to have the view that the balance of power is too much in favour of women. On balance, though, these groups do believe that men get a better deal than women.

Separated or divorced men are less likely to feel men are in the better situation; their lower score suggests that the divorce courts tend to make a man feel downtrodden. Correspondingly, they are much less likely than married, cohabiting or single men to say men have too much power in Britain today, and 18 per cent say women have the better deal.

Men without a relationship are less inclined to say men have the upper hand, as are those who've only had one partner.

MEN ON SEX

Rich men – those earning over £25k – are more likely than the lower earners to say women have the best deal. The unemployed are also more inclined than most to feel women have the best deal.

Men on Top

Cohabitors are particularly likely to say men get the best of the bargain. The type of relationships a man has seems to affect his view of male versus female supremacy. Meanwhile, the two-timers – those having their cake and eating it – are among the most likely to say men have the advantage. They should know!

Eighteen per cent of disillusioned separated men, but only 4 per cent of men with no relationship and none of the two-timers, think women are on top in Britain today.

Power Struggle

The more education a man has had, the more likely he is to say the balance of power is too much in favour of men. This stance, which could be interpreted as a feminist statement, is also more likely to be taken up by men in their late 30s, the unemployed and those who lost their virginity late. Men with very young children are less likely to hold this view, although the older their children get, the more liberal they become: only 44 per cent of men with children under the age of four say men have too much power, compared with 60 per cent of those living with children aged ten and above.

The more basic his education and lower his type of employment, the more likely a man is to think that the balance of power is about right. By contrast, far fewer of the unemployed say the situation is ideal.

Only 20 per cent of men sometimes find it difficult to express their views in female company for fear of being accused of sexism. Separated men have a higher than average score here, while none of the two-timers or men with very young children feel this is a big problem. However, men who never have sex are more likely to feel inhibited in the presence of women. Those who find this a ridiculous idea are more likely to earn over £25k, to be separated or to have children under four.

WHAT'S MY LINE?

According to the majority of men in our survey, it makes little difference to them whether it's a man or woman driving their bus or train, operating on them, defending them in court or representing them in Parliament. This represents a huge change in prevailing social attitudes since the 60s, or even the 70s, when feminism was beginning to bite, but was largely dismissed by men as irrelevant. Even ten years ago, there was no question that driving a bus was a man's job. And now? This table shows which sex men would prefer to work for them in the following professions.

MALE OR FEMALE?

	MAN	WOMAN	NO DIFFERENCE	DON'T KNOW
Bus/Train driver	24%	1%	73%	2%
Doctor	25%	9%	63%	3%
Surgeon	24%	2%	72%	3%
Lawyer	22%	5%	70%	3%
MP	16%	2%	80%	2%

Men find the idea of a woman doctor more acceptable than females in the other roles, and are particularly willing to agree that the sex of their MP makes no difference.

Highly educated men are less likely than most to have a preference for male surgeons or doctors. However, the men in the middle education range are the strongest supporters of equality in the House of Commons: 86 per cent of them say the sex of their MP is irrelevant. Those who have a limited education are more likely to prefer a male doctor, train or bus driver.

The youngest men find the idea of a woman defending them in court much more acceptable than the oldest group; 9 per cent would prefer a female lawyer, compared with just 3 per cent of men over 40. Men aged 18-24 also like the idea of a female doctor more than the older generation: 16 per cent are in favour of a woman GP, whereas only 5 per cent of men over 40 would actively seek out a female doctor.

Men over 40 are also more likely than most to prefer having a man than a woman wielding a scalpel near them. Those in their

MEN ON SEX

late 20s, however, are the most likely to say the sex of their surgeon is of no importance to them.

The pattern of youth and liberal attitudes is reversed, though, when it comes to bus and train drivers. Here, having a man in the driving seat is more important to young men than to those who left their train sets behind a long time ago.

The amount a man earns has little effect on his opinion of which sex makes the best lawyers or surgeons. But there are differences for the other professions. Lower earners are more likely than those with higher salaries to prefer a female doctor, while men earning over £25k are more likely to say it makes no difference who drives their bus or train, or represents them in Parliament.

Men in lower forms of employment tend to prefer male surgeons, doctors, train and bus drivers. The unemployed, meanwhile, come out strongly in favour of female lawyers, surgeons and doctors, but are more likely than average to want a man as an MP, train or bus driver.

Having had a greater number of partners seems to make a man more inclined to choose a woman in these professions. Seven per cent of men who've had more than ten partners would prefer a female lawyer, against just 2 per cent of men who've only had one partner. There's a similar pattern in their preference for surgeons, doctors and MPs.

Men who have sex most often are also more likely than those with less charged sex lives to prefer women lawyers and surgeons. However, 34 per cent of men who have sex at least four times a week feel happier with a male doctor, compared with just 25 per cent, on average.

MAN'S BEST FRIEND

The picture changed quite dramatically when we asked whether men would rather have a male or female as their best friend.

MALE OR FEMALE?			
MAN	WOMAN	NO DIFFERENCE	DON'T KNOW
31%	17%	48%	4%

At this point, men are much more conscious of sex, and far fewer say that it makes no difference.

Less than a third of men would insist on their best friend being a man. Having a male best friend is much more important to those with a regular relationship than it is for the two-timers: 36 per cent of men with a bit on the side would also prefer their best friend to be a woman. Married men rate male best friends more highly than separated men. Divorced or separated men go against the usual pattern in our sample: 22 per cent would prefer a man and 28 per cent would choose a woman, while 51 per cent say it makes no difference. Men with occasional relationships also split their vote more evenly between men and women as friends.

Those notably more likely than most to say a best mate must be a man include those in their late 20s and the unemployed.

SELLING ON SEX

When we asked men whether they thought sex in advertising is demeaning to women, only a quarter agreed. Many more – 37 per cent of men – were inclined to disagree, 24 per cent stayed neutral and 14 per cent didn't know what to think on this issue. Separated men had the strongest views here, with 38 per cent saying that sex in advertising *does* degrade women. However, a massive 58 per cent of two-timers think it's a ridiculous idea – the more sex, the better! Men having sex more than four times a week also tend to agree with them.

This question provoked a few unexpected complaints that *men* are exploited by advertising. A single 21 year old from the Yorkshire/Humberside area said: 'I feel males are put under a lot of pressure – equal to or even more so than females – because of the way they are portrayed in advertising and other media.' A cohabiting 26 year old from the North East put forward the New Man's point of view: 'A major problem I find about sex is that the mass media tends to portray the "macho" side, rather than the sensual, caring side which sex should be a manifestation of.'

In line with their view that sex as a selling point isn't demeaning to women, almost half the men in our sample disagree that men want less sex in advertising. A quarter sit on the fence and only 10 per cent agree that men are tired of sexy adverts. As before, it's the men having the most sex who most oppose the idea of cutting down on sex in adverts, while men who lost their virginity relatively late are among the most likely to say men would like to cut down on sex in advertising.

DEEP IN THE WOODS

And, finally, to Iron John. This American movement, based on Robert Bly's book *Iron John*, is the latest in consciousness-raising for men. It's definitely for warriors, not wimps, and involves a good deal of running about wooded areas getting back to basic emotions – wild men in wild places. The New Man tried to fit the image of the perfect man according to feminist ideals. But Iron John rejects this 'emasculation' by women. Instead, the movement aims to encourage men to express their emotions and resolve the conflicts that exist between fathers and sons.

We wanted to find out if men in our sample thought their relationship with their father had been a great influence on how they felt about being a man. Their answers were fairly noncommittal.

MY FATHER INFLUENCED THE WAY I FEEL ABOUT BEING A MAN	
Strongly agree	8%
Tend to agree	22%
Neither	25%
Tend to disagree	19%
Strongly disagree	18%
Don't know	8%

As only 8 per cent think their fathers *did* have a profound effect on their self-image, it seems that only a very few men in our sample would be interested in attending an Iron John weekend!

Perhaps the reason why so few men consider their fathers a great influence is because fathers generally have a less active role than mothers in bringing up children. Or it could be that they see little comparison between their fathers' masculinity and their own. They may feel that example no longer applies to masculine and feminine roles today. If a man grows up in a household where his mother is not allowed to have a cheque book, let alone a job, he may not find his father's behaviour a useful role model for life with an independent working wife or girlfriend.

One single 18 year old from the East Midlands was in no doubt that his father had had no influence whatsoever on him: 'I've never seen the bastard and I feel I've grown up a better person because of that!' However, separated men are much more likely than the rest to think their father did influence how they feel about being a man. Fifteen per cent strongly agree with the statement and 30 per cent tend to agree with it, as do 31 per cent of the two-timers.

Men in our sample obviously find it easier to take some 'feminist' ideas on board than others. In most cases, a clear majority accept there is no difference between men and women in the professional arena, two-thirds say men still get the best deal, and over half believe men have too much power in Britain today. Almost half get a (masculine) kick from sport, and few like the idea of cutting down on sex in advertising. Of the two male figures supposedly closest to a man – his father and his best friend – one is rejected as a strong influence and the other can be a woman! So it's hardly surprising that as social and sexual attitudes are changing, there's conflict and confusion over 'masculine' territory.

2.

A Question of Priorities

We asked all the men in our sample to consider what mattered most to them in life. Here are the twenty most frequently mentioned items, with the percentage of men who expressed an interest in each.

WHAT REALLY MATTERS TO MEN?

THE TOP 20

1.	Job satisfaction	52%	11. Car	33%
2.	Partner	46%	=12. Job security	32%
3.	Home	43%	=12. Having a job	32%
4.	Independence	39%	14. Sex	31%
5.	Freedom	38%	=15. Appearance	30%
= 6.	Career	36%	=15. Peace and quiet	30%
= 6.	Health	36%	17. Children	29%
= 6.	Leisure/hobbies	36%	18. Female friends	27%
9.	Social life	35%	19. Male friends	26%
10.	Money	34%	20. Holidays abroad	22%

Job Satisfaction

Given that they spend an average of more than 43 hours a week at work (i.e. half their waking life), it's hardly surprising that job satisfaction is the one factor mentioned by more than half the sample. Its importance is most marked in men in their late 30s (it becomes less important in the 40s), and applies across all educational and income levels. It's not linked with how sexually active a man is, though it is less important to men who have had the most sexual partners. It's also less important to men in the South of England than those in the North.

Partner

Men's second concern is their partner. Partners are particularly important to older men, and are rated highest among married men and lowest among those who are separated, higher among fathers than non fathers, and particularly high among those who live together but don't have children. Not surprisingly, men who have remained faithful to their first sexual partner rate her particularly highly, while those who have had more than ten sexual partners tend to rate their current partner less highly. Those who are having the most sex (at least four times a week) are most interested in their partners.

Home

The third most highly rated concern is home. This is particularly true for older men and for those with less education, though it's not related to income level. Men currently separated from their partners are particularly interested in their home, though it's not clear whether this reflects nostalgia for a home they no longer have or pleasure in creating a new one.

Independence and Freedom

Next on the list come the psychological variables independence and freedom. Both are particularly important to the young and much less important to men over 35. Men earning less than £15k a year value freedom and independence more than higher earners, as do those with occasional relationships or none at all.

> MEN ON SEX

Career, Health and Leisure

Researchers have argued about the relative importance to men of work and leisure. The men in our sample rate them as equally important. In fact there's a three-way tie between them and health for the sixth most important concern in men's lives. Single men and non-fathers rate having a career more highly than those with partners or children. As income level rises and men get older, it seems to become less important to have a career. Similarly, interest in leisure activities and hobbies tends to decline after 35 and therefore with income status. There is no link between educational level and leisure. Men without children have more time for leisure activities. Interest in health seems to have little to do with age, nor is it linked with marital status or having children. The less well educated and low-income groups are particularly interested in health, as are two-timers, i.e. men with both a regular relationship and another partner.

Social Life

Not surprisingly, the younger a man is, the more important it is for him to have a good social life. The higher his education and income, the less important it becomes. A good social life is particularly important both to those who have very little sex (less than once a month or never) and to those who are having a great deal, though the two groups may have very different reasons for socialising. A good social life is also rated more highly in the North than in other parts of the country.

Money

Money just scrapes into the Top Ten and is of particular importance to men under 24. Men with good jobs are very interested in money, but so are the unemployed. Married men are less interested in money than those who are single or cohabiting. Fathers are also less concerned with the subject than men without children.

Car

Young men aged 18-24, single men, and those earning less than £15k are most keen on having a car.

Job

Job security and having a job hold equal twelfth place, and are much greater concerns for people with basic education and a lower income than for men with higher education and those earning over £25k.

Sex

This doesn't even make it into the Top Ten, and the fact that it comes eleven places lower in the list than 'partner' throws an interesting light on the real reasons behind the traditional male preoccupation with sex. Young lads under 24 are more interested in sex than most, as are those with basic education, an income below £15k, men in higher forms of employment, and those seeking work. Cohabitors are much more interested in sex than married men – a finding confirmed by their higher levels of sexual activity (see Chapter Four). Being a father has no effect on a man's preoccupation with sex. Only 10 per cent of men without a relationship are concerned with sex, compared with a massive 61 per cent of the two-timers, for whom it is by far the highest priority on their list! Generally, the more sex a man has and the more partners he's had, the more important he rates sex. A disposition towards sex is also linked to losing your virginity early and enjoying it a great deal the first time. So it seems safe to accept that a preoccupation with sex is a genuine personality trait.

Appearance

Men rate their physical appearance pretty highly, although there's no place in the Top Twenty for clothes. Younger men, the lower earners, single men and those without children are most concerned with how they look. Of all the groups, two-timing men rate their appearance least important. Yet the more partners a man's had, the more he values his looks. We can only speculate as to what lies behind this. Perhaps having to attend to two women simultaneously leaves little time for a man to preen himself, while the need to make ever more sexual conquests can be seen as a sign of excessive vanity or a need to be continually reassured, either (or both) of which might also be manifested in frequent glances at the mirror.

MEN ON SEX

Peace and Quiet

Men over 40 and those earning over £25k value peace and quiet – at their age, maybe they think they've earned it. Separated men also feel peace and quiet are important; two-timers by contrast are least interested in the quiet life!

Children

Children are particularly important to men over 35 and to the higher earners. For men living with children, this interest declines gradually as their children get older. Men having sex four times a week and those having it less than once a month are not as interested in their children as those having a moderate amount of sex.

Friends

Having good female friends is most important to the 18-24 year olds and men earning up to £15k. They are also more important to separated and single men, non fathers and people with occasional relationships. Interestingly, it is these groups who are also likely to rate their male friends as important, but less so than their female friends. Men having sex less than once a month value female friends particularly highly, while it's those having sex four times a week who say male companions are more important.

Holidays Abroad

People living together without children and non fathers are among those most likely to say holidaying abroad is important to them.

Lower Priorities

A few more interesting priorities emerged after the first 20, and these were parents, clothes, power, politics and religion.

Just one in five men say their parents are particularly important to them. Parents are a higher priority for men with basic education and those earning less than £15k. The fewer partners a man has had, the more likely it is he rates his parents highly, while separated men give their parents a lower priority than people who are living together or single. Men who are themselves living with young children seem to value their own parents more highly, perhaps because they value their advice or maybe because they have a new understanding of them!

Clothes hold most appeal for young men under 24, people with basic education and those earning up to £15k. Single men and those without children also have more interest in what they wear. Fashion designer Paul Costelloe is not surprised that clothes are such a low priority for men today: 'British men still look at clothes as functional. Fashion is irrelevant.' He also feels it's an attitude specific to this country, and one that does nothing for men's sex appeal. 'The main problem with British males is British females who put them in school uniform from the time they're little boys. English men can look brilliant, but most of them don't know how to wear adventurous clothes in a masculine way. Conventional men's tailoring can be smart, but you can't make men sexy like that. John Major's a classic example, he tucks his shirt into his underpants – that's the end. But you can't change him, it's too late. I hate British men wearing V-neck jumpers – they're sexlessness personified, so are cravats and Barbours. They say "I'm a British chap", there's no mystery.'

Power and politics came near the end of the list (tying with 9 per cent each), while religion trails last with only 8 per cent. Power interests men earning over £25k, and those in higher forms of employment. Men with ten or more partners and those having sex four times a week or more are also more likely to be interested in power. It is linked to early, unenjoyable loss of virginity. These findings appear to support the notion that power is an aphrodisiac rather than another popular theory, that men who pursue power are seeking compensation for sexual inadequacy. It's not difficult to see why men who enjoy feeling powerful would be turned off by their first sexual encounter. Fathers with children under four, by contrast, have virtually no interest in it.

Politics appeals most to men in their early 30s. Those having a lot of sex and those who never do are more interested in politics than the regular sex guys, while two-timers are not at all likely to be political animals.

It is not surprising that religion is most important to men with only one partner, those who lost their virginity late and men who never have sex. This clustering seems to indicate another personality type: the non-sexual person. A single man in his early 40s, living in London, makes the connection between religion and celibacy: 'I feel that I am a holy man and that I have no use for testicles whatsoever.' There are higher percentages of believers among the unemployed, while separated men and two-timers seem particularly disenchanted with religion.

GETTING THE HABIT

So much for what men think about most. But what do they actually *do,* and what do they feel about themselves?

We also asked men to tell us about their lifestyle, diet and habits. The results are striking. Fifty-seven per cent of our sample said they take part in sport or exercise on a regular basis. It's most popular with men under 30, those with medium levels of education and people earning £15-25k. Men without children are more likely to take exercise than fathers, and two-timing men are particularly keen on sport. The more sex you have, the more likely it is you practise sport, and the men who've had two to nine partners are more likely to exercise than those who've had either one partner or more than nine. So another popular myth bites the dust: taking violent exercise is *not* a sex substitute!

Two out of five men eat fast food – a habit that goes with youth, lower earnings and unemployment. Single men, non fathers and men having sex more than four times a week also like fast food.

Twenty-seven per cent of the men in our sample smoke cigarettes. The habit is most widespread among the young, those with basic and medium levels of education and lower earners. Interestingly, separated men are much more likely to smoke than married, cohabiting or single men. The more partners you've had, the more likely it is you smoke, and the men having sex more than four times a week are also keen on cigarettes. Evidence here perhaps of an addictive personality at work? Men who lose their virginity late are cautious about smoking, and are four times less likely to be smokers than those who lost it early. Caution is clearly another personality trait that affects many aspects of behaviour.

Nine per cent of our sample diet to lose weight, particularly the older men, those earning more and in higher forms of employment. Men who have sex less than once a month and those with no current relationship are less likely to be cutting down on their intake of calories.

The men in our sample are more likely to smoke dope (7 per cent) than a pipe or cigars (3 per cent). The dope smokers tend to be younger men under 24, those earning less than £15k and the unemployed. Cohabiting and single men are much more likely to indulge in marijuana than those who are married or separated. Other fans of this type of weed include the highly sexually active, those having sex less than once a month, men who've had ten or more partners and people who lost their virginity early. Only 1 per cent of our sample takes cocaine, and the same small percentage uses aphrodisiacs.

IN THERAPY

What about other physical and mental balms? We asked men what use they make of various types of therapy currently available. A quarter of them have had a massage, particularly men in higher employment. It's linked to a lot of sexual activity, having had a lot of partners and losing your virginity early. By contrast, men without relationships have little experience of massage.

There is a three-way tie for the second most popular form of therapy, between homeopathy, psychotherapy/psychoanalysis and yoga – though each has been tried by only one man in twenty in our sample. The over 40s are particularly keen on homeopathy, and more of them have also experienced psychotherapy and psychoanalysis, along with 18 per cent of the separated men. Men who lost their virginity early and those who've had more than ten partners are also more likely to have had psychotherapy. By contrast, none of the two-timers is drawn towards such introspective activity. Yoga is slightly more popular with the over 40s and those with higher education; it also appeals to 10 per cent of men who never have sex.

Four per cent have had recourse to marriage counselling; of these 29 people, it's most common among the older, more affluent men, those with higher education, and men with better jobs. Predictably, separated men are the most likely to have tried it. Acupuncture is also used by 4 per cent of the sample and again, it is the older, better educated men with a higher income who are likely to be devotees. Married men, two-timers and men with more than ten partners are also keen on the treatment. Three per cent of our men are keen on aromatherapy – it's particularly popular with separated men and those with more than ten partners. Amongst men with only one partner, however, its use is unknown. The Alexander Technique and sex therapy score 1 per cent each.

Perhaps the most telling comment on the state of mind of our sample comes from the finding that almost two-thirds of them have no experience of *any* of these forms of therapy!

ROLE MODELS?

The impression of contentment given by the statistics above is confirmed by the results of another probe we used to get a fix on them. We gave them a list of sixteen successful public figures, from a number of different fields, and asked them which they admired. The list below is interesting, not least for the fact that only one public figure attracted more votes than the response indicating that *none* of the men named was a figure of admiration!

MEN I ADMIRE	
Richard Branson	25%
Gary Lineker	20%
Robin Williams	14%
Nigel Mansell	13%
Arnold Schwarzenegger	8%
Alan Sugar	7%
Lenny Henry	6%
Prince Charles	4%
Ben Elton	4%
Mel Gibson	4%
Lord Hanson	4%
Mick Jagger	3%
Jeremy Paxman	2%
Jonathon Porritt	2%
Melvyn Bragg	1%
Rupert Murdoch	1%
None of these	23%

Richard Branson appeals most to older men, those with better jobs and men earning over £25k. He's liked least by single men. In the discussion groups, he was admired as a man who challenges the establishment, is courageous and unconventional. 'I like Branson because he always tries something that appears to be out of the ordinary. I admire that – I'd like to be able to do that,' said a married 41 year old. The feeling was that he had worked his way up and achieved results through his own merit: 'He has come from working in the shed at the bottom of the garden to building up something quite special,' said a cohabiting 25 year old. The reality of Branson's rise to success may be somewhat different, but the men's perception is all that matters.

Men with ten partners or more are least likely to have marked the box 'None of these', while men who never have sex are more likely to say they don't identify with any of the men listed. In the small group discussions, a married 35 year old explained his reservations about men who've made it: 'I tend to have the feeling that successful men have got to their position of success by being perhaps unpleasant, perhaps stepping on others to get there. Which is not admirable. So, there are many people I know who I admire, but not many in public life.'

Gary Lineker gained votes from the over 40s, separated men and the unemployed, while those who never have sex gave him a particularly low score. Men in the discussion groups clearly admired Lineker as a well-mannered footballer who believes in fair play. His new baby also gained him extra points. A married 35 year old said: 'Lineker's in the situation of being a role model, and he performs that very well. He's also got a bit to say for himself when he's interviewed.'

Young single men with a lower income like Robin Williams, but married men and two-timers rate him less highly. Nigel Mansell is a hero for the over 40s, but not for cohabitors or people living with very young children. Among those who attracted less than 10 per cent, Arnold Schwarzenegger appeals to the young, low earners, the unemployed and people with occasional relationships. He's twice as popular with men without children as with fathers, and those who lost their virginity early also admire him. Men in higher forms of employment and those earning over £25k think more highly of Alan Sugar and Lord Hanson. Lenny Henry is most popular with men in their early 30s, while Prince Charles has more fans among men who never have sex than any other group! Men over 35 are not at all keen on Ben Elton, although the unemployed like him. Mel Gibson gains votes from

| MEN ON SEX | the 18-24 year olds, while Mick Jagger has no support from the men who never have sex. Jeremy Paxman has support from those in higher employment and the two-timers. Jonathon Porritt can console himself that of the 2 per cent who admire him, the majority are the over 40s, the higher educated, men earning over £25k and those in higher forms of employment.

It seems that politicians and priests have little influence in men's lives, and few of the public figures on our list inspire hero worship. Action, in the form of sport, beats reflection, in the form of psychoanalysis: exercise has a role to play for 57 per cent, while only 5 per cent have experience of the analyst's couch. It's also telling that freedom and independence are of more value than sex or money. But for the men in our sample, the bare necessities of life closest to their hearts are their jobs, their partners and their homes.

3.

First Bite at the Cherry

Sex may not be an all-consuming passion for men, but it's certainly a subject that interests them. So when does it all begin? In our sample, 16 or 17 are by far the most common ages for a man to lose his virginity, and the more partners he has had, the more likely this is.

Many men in the small group discussions described losing their virginity as a major milestone in their development and proof they'd reached adulthood. A married 35 year old confirmed the significance of getting it over with by the age of 16: 'At our school we were all approaching our 16th birthdays and it was like, anyone who reaches 16 and he's still a virgin – what a nancy!' This kind of male peer-group pressure seemed to be a common factor for men in the groups. Telling your friends was a vital part of the experience, and no-one would have lost their virginity without mentioning it. There was a feeling, however, that some may have lied and said they'd had sex when they hadn't.

The table overleaf shows when men in our sample first had sex.

A significant minority of the men in our sample started sexual activity illegally young: one man in five had his first experience of sexual intercourse before the age of consent (16). Those most likely to have lost their virginity before the age of 14 have a number of distinguishing characteristics: they are the men with more than ten partners and those who have sex four or more times a week. Cohabitors are also three times as likely as married men to have lost their virginity before they were 14.

Men who've had more than five partners, those having sex four times a week and the two-timers are particularly likely to

SEX BEGINS AT...

Age	%
Less than 14	4%
14-15	16%
16-17	31%
18-19	23%
20-21	10%
22-24	5%
25-29	2%
30-39	<1%
40+	<1%
Can't remember	2%
Never had sex	5%

have lost their virginity aged 14 or 15. Men who first have sex at this age are more likely than most to have a basic level of education; by contrast, men with a higher level of education are more likely to have lost their virginity at the comparatively late age of 20-21.

A third of the men who've only ever had one partner lost their virginity aged 18-19, compared with 23 per cent on average, while all but one of the men in our sample who've had more than ten partners lost their virginity before they were 25. Unsurprisingly, the older men in our sample lost their virginity later than young men do today.

Eleven per cent of the youngest age group – the men under 24 – have never had sex. As you'd expect, this figure drops dramatically with age: 7 per cent of 25-29 year olds are virgins, 2 per cent of 30-34 year olds, none of the 35-39 year olds and just 1 per cent of 40-45 year olds. A single 26 year old from the South East pointed out that some people may want to save sex for marriage, and complained that there was no provision in our questionnaire for men to say 'I don't believe in pre-marital sex'.

So much for the age at which sexual initiation took place. But what actually happened, who else was involved, and how do our men remember feeling afterwards?

Fifty-six per cent of the men lost their virginity to somebody they knew well; 30 per cent first had sex with someone they knew a little, and for 14 per cent, the partner was someone they had just met! Married men and those over 40 are the most likely to have lost their virginity to somebody they knew well, as are men who first had sex relatively late. Two-timers, on the other hand, are more likely to have gone for someone they knew only a little. Men who've had ten or more partners are more likely than men in the other groups to have first had sex with someone they had just met, and are the *least* likely to have lost their virginity to someone they knew well. Men who lost their virginity later are, on the other hand, much more likely to have been with someone they knew well.

We asked the 749 men who've had sexual intercourse about the circumstances in which they lost their virginity. They are described in the following table.

HOW WAS IT FOR YOU?

We didn't use contraception	35%
I was in love	24%
We planned the occasion	21%
It was a one-night stand	17%
I was at a party	13%
My parents were away	12%
My then partner's parents were away	12%
I was drunk	11%
I was on holiday	8%
I'd been taking drugs	2%
I was with a prostitute	1%
None of these	14%

For most of our men, the first time seems to have been a chaotic occasion. More than a third of them first experienced sex unprotected by contraception. ' I bet the number who ticked "we didn't use contraception" was high. Now I sweat! I think, my God, I was so lucky!' said a cohabiting 39 year old in one of the groups. Men with basic education, those who are separated and the unemployed are the people most likely not to have used contraception. Fathers are more likely than non fathers not to have used contraception the first time – which may explain why they have children now! Men without a relationship are more likely than two-timers not to have taken precautions. Men who lost their virginity early and those who have had a lot of partners are particularly unlikely to have used contraception for their first sexual experience.

Fifty-four per cent of the men who have only ever had one partner say they were in love when they lost their virginity, compared with only 12 per cent of men who've had ten or more partners. Men in lower forms of employment are much more likely to say they were in love, as are cohabiting men and late starters, whereas single men and those who have the most sex are less likely to say they were in love. Those who were in love are more likely to say they enjoyed the first time, as are those men who say they had planned the occasion. So much for careless rapture!

The over 40s and the unemployed are unlikely to have planned the loss of their virginity, whereas men who've had only one partner and those who have sex four or more times a week are more likely to have done so. One comment on the idea of a planned occasion, 'I would have liked to see the inclusion of a category "I was celebrating my wedding",' came from a married 26 year old from the South East.

Losing your virginity on a one-night stand is more common among the young, single men, those who start having sex early and men who've had five plus partners. It's much less common among two-timers. Moreover, according to men in our survey, one-night stands are a poor recipe for enjoying your first sexual experience.

Losing your virginity at a party is particularly common among the unemployed and single men. The more sexual partners a man has had, the more likely it is that he first had sex at a party.

Men having sex four times or more a week are much more likely than those who currently never have sex to have taken advantage of their partner's parents being away. However, these men are much less likely to have selected their own home as a venue for their deflowering.

The men most likely to say that they were drunk at the time are those aged 18-24, those earning less than £15k, and the unemployed. Other inebriated sexual initiates are likely to be single rather than married and without children. Being drunk when losing your virginity also seems more likely to lead to an unpleasant experience!

Seventeen per cent of men currently without a relationship lost their virginity on holiday. This is much more common for the married and single men than for cohabitors or those who are separated. Separated and single men are the most likely to have taken drugs; 6 per cent of 18-24 year olds also come into this category. Nine per cent of the men who never have sex at the moment had taken drugs when they lost their virginity. The 1 per cent whose first experience of sex was with a prostitute tend to belong to the group of separated men.

ENJOYING THE EXPERIENCE

We asked men how much they enjoyed sex when they lost their virginity. The pattern of their replies isn't affected by age, education, income or employment. Only one man in four says he enjoyed the experience a lot. Another 36 per cent liked it quite a lot, but almost as many men enjoyed it only a little, not very much or not at all (7 per cent of our sample say they can't remember how they felt). Men in the discussion groups didn't feel that their subsequent sex life has been affected by how much they enjoyed losing their virginity. 'At 16 or 17, it's a flash in the pan. You go on to your next conquest,' said one married 35 year old. Separated men and those with occasional relationships are most likely to say they enjoyed losing their virginity a great deal. Men who have sex four times a week or more and those who have sex less than once a month are also more likely than other groups to say they enjoyed the first time.

Men who've had only one partner, those who have sex less than once a month and men who lost their virginity late are all particularly likely to say they enjoyed it a fair amount. Two-timers are less likely than the rest to say they didn't have a good time, and none of them say they didn't enjoy the experience at all. However, in the discussion groups, a cohabiting 39 year old described the horrors of losing his virginity: 'For me it was a smutty furtive affair in which I was lucky to get a stiffy, as they say. An absolute anticlimax and I thought, if this is what it's like, forget it, pal! Just the memory of it makes me weep!'

THE VENUE

As for venue, the following table shows where men in our survey had their first taste of sex.

SEX ON LOCATION

Bedroom	58%
Living-room	15%
Car	6%
Outdoors in the country	6%
Outdoors elsewhere	5%
Beach/seaside	2%
Tent/caravan	2%
Bathroom	2%
Kitchen	1%
Other room in the house	1%
Place of work	1%
Other	3%

The men most likely to have made it to the bedroom are the 25-34 year olds, those with higher education and men earning £15-£25k. The two-timers are the least likely to have lost their virginity in bed. The later a man lost his virginity, the more likely it is to have happened in the bedroom. This venue is also linked with greater enjoyment of sex the first time.

The living-room was a common choice for the over 40s and was more usual for fathers than non fathers. The over 40s also liked in-car sex more than most, as did the cohabitors and two-timers. Ten per cent of men who've only had one partner lost their virginity in the back of a car. Sex outside in the countryside also held an appeal for the over 40s and for separated men. Losing your virginity in the open air is three times as likely for men who started early as for those who first had sex aged 16-19. Those with basic education, men earning up to £15k and the unemployed are more likely to have picked some other outdoor site, as are the men who started early. The early starters are also slightly more likely to have discovered the joys of sex beside the seaside.

Some of the comments written on questionnaires suggested that a few men had first experienced sex in more unusual circumstances, such as the man who lost his virginity in a mud hut in Angola with a prostitute. Other locations cited were the school laundry-room, a telephone box, the woods, on a boat, on a golf course and in a swimming pool.

Over half the men in our sample chose a partner they knew well, and the results show that love, rather than alcohol, was the secret for enjoying the occasion. Although a minority couldn't remember exactly when they lost their virginity, for most it was a memorable landmark on the way to adulthood. However, for around a third of our men, the event was an anti-climax. Predictably, the bedroom proved a more popular venue for first-night performances than a boat or beach hut, but the last word must go to the man who explains how he came to lose his virginity both outdoors and in a bedroom: 'Had to finish inside due to weather!'

4.

The Numbers Game

Less than one man in five in our sample has confined his sexual experience to a single partner – though more than two-thirds of them have done so over the last 12 months. However, almost 70 per cent have limited their sexual liaisons to single figures, with only one man in ten having had 20 or more sexual partners.

HOW MANY?

HOW MANY – EVER?	
PARTNER(S)	
1	18%
2-4	27%
5-9	24%
10-14	10%
15-19	5%
20-29	3%
More than 30	7%
Can't remember	7%

Men who've only ever had one partner are more likely to be married or cohabiting, to be in lower forms of employment, or to have children under the age of four. The age at which a man loses his virginity is another factor: 37 per cent of late starters have only had one partner, compared with just 5 per cent of early starters. Men who never have sex these days are also extremely likely only to have had one partner: 39 per cent of these men come into this category, compared with just 12 per cent of men who have sex more than four times a week.

A married 26 year old from the South East was a staunch advocate of monogamy: 'I am concerned and disappointed that this view is unrepresented, i.e. one woman being the most important person and only life-time sex partner for a man in the 90s. Numerous discussions over a number of years have shown me that this idea is one that many men would like to achieve as a way of communicating to a woman how special she is.'

The youngest group – the 18-24 year olds – are the most likely to have had two to four partners. This is probably because they are too young to have had a great number of partners, which also explains the higher percentages of single men, those without children and men without relationships who come into this category. Many more of those who lost their virginity relatively late have also restricted themselves to one sexual partner; as this table shows, men who postpone their sexual initiation until later are more likely to opt for monogamy than other men in our sample.

MEN WHO'VE HAD ONE SEXUAL PARTNER

AGE OF LOSS OF VIRGINITY

Under 15	5%
16-19	16%
20 or over	37%

Many of the married, single and unemployed men have had sexual liaisons with five to nine partners. However, the over 40s are likely to have had fewer partners, and those who are separated tend to claim either fewer, or many more than this figure! Men who have sex more than four times a week, or once a week, are also represented among those who have had between five and

MEN ON SEX

nine partners, as are men who lost their virginity early rather than late, and those who didn't enjoy it the first time.

By the time we reach 10-14 partners, the percentages of all groups drop significantly. Men aged 30-34 are well represented, as are higher earners, fathers and those with regular or occasional relationships. Interestingly, men having the most sex tend not to have had as many partners: the majority of highly sexually active men have had between one and nine partners. This may be partly explained by the higher number of young men who have the most sex.

Of the 5 per cent of men who claim 15-19 partners, many tend to have one or more of the following characteristics: aged over 35, medium levels of education, higher forms of employment, separated. Those who lay claim to 20-29 partners tend to be in their late 20s; two-timers and early starters are also represented in this group.

As the first table showed, 7 per cent of the sexually experienced men in our sample have had more than 30 partners, and these men tend to be aged over 35. Men who've had more than 30 partners also tend to have an income over £25k, high-status jobs, and to be separated. Two-timers are also represented in this category.

The men who say they can't remember how many people they've had sex with are likely to have basic education, a lower income and a lower status job. The earlier you start having sex, the more likely it is that you've lost count! Men in occasional relationships also seem prone to forgetfulness – and a staggering 21 per cent of two-timers suffer from selective amnesia when it comes to counting the score in this area.

ANNUAL REPORT

So much for life-time numbers. But how many sexual partners have our men had over the past 12 months?

The great majority of our sample have confined themselves to a single partner in the last year. This is particularly so in the 35-39 age group and among higher earners. Eighty-five per cent of married men and 82 per cent of cohabitors have stayed with one partner in the past 12 months. As you would expect, men with fewer partners are generally more likely to come into this category, as are those who have sex once a week or less. The later he lost his virginity, the more likely it is that a man will have been faithful to one sexual partner in the last year.

HOW MANY – LAST YEAR?	
PARTNER(S)	
1	68%
2-4	16%
5-9	3%
10-14	1%
15-19	–
20-29	1%
30+	1%
None	3%
Can't remember	7%

Men who have had 2-4 partners in the last year are more likely to be under 24, less well paid and perhaps even unemployed. Men who have sex less than once a month and those who lost their virginity early rather than late are also well represented among those who have had two to four partners in the last year, as are singles, separated men and those in occasional relationships. No less than half the two-timers fall into this category.

Men who have had five to nine partners over the same period tend to have the following characteristics: basic education, and early loss of virginity. Only one married man in a 100 has had sex with this many partners in the past year – a reassuring thought for wives – compared with the 9 per cent of separated men who lay claim to this hit-rate. Only 1 per cent of our sample claim to have slept with 10-14 partners in the past year, i.e. an average of one new person a month.

As before, 7 per cent of our men can't remember how many partners they've had in the last year. They are most likely to be those who lost their virginity early and enjoyed it, and those with basic education. A fair proportion of the two-timers and those without a current relationship have also lost count of their partners over the past 12 months.

HOW OFTEN?

As for frequency, 13 per cent have sex at least four times a week (with one man in 50 making it a daily occurrence). At the other extreme, almost a third have sex only once a fortnight or less often. The most common pattern seems to be sex two or three times a week.

HOW OFTEN?

Every day or more than once a day	2%
4-6 times a week	11%
2-3 times a week	33%
Once a week	19%
Once a fortnight	11%
Once a month	7%
Less than once a month	13%
Never, at present	5%

NB: These figures apply to the non-virgins in the sample.

Broadly speaking, the more sexual partners a man has had in the past, the more frequently he will be having sex today. Daily sex is more likely for men who lost their virginity early.

Having sex four to six times a week is linked to basic rather than higher education, and lower rather than higher income. Again, cohabitors have sex much more frequently than single, separated or married men. Young men under 30 are the most likely to have sex four to six times a week. Those non-parents living with a partner are three times more likely to enjoy this level of sexual activity than men living with young children. The earlier a man loses his virginity, the more likely it is he has sex four to six times a week now. Two-timers are also well represented here.

A third of the men in our sample have sex two to three times a week. The groups most likely to have this amount of sexual activity are men in their late 30s, those earning over £25k, married men and fathers. Half of the two-timers come into this category, as do a third of men who've had more than ten partners and a third of men with regular relationships. Men who have sex two to three times a week are more likely to have lost their virginity between the ages of 16 and 19, but to have enjoyed the experience only a little.

Once a week men are likely to be old rather than young, and to have higher levels of education. Married men and fathers are also inclined to have sex on a weekly basis, particularly if they have young children (whereas men with older children are more likely to have sex two or three times a week).

The once-a-fortnight pattern is commoner among older men, particularly those in their late 30s. This pattern of sexual activity is also associated with a medium level of education and employment, and the middle income bracket (£15k-£25k). Fifteen per cent of married men have sex twice a month.

Seven per cent of all non-virgins in our sample now have sex once a month. Men in their late 30s are least likely to come into this category. It is however a pattern found among cohabitors, single men and those with occasional relationships. Men who are single and those who have occasional relationships are also over-represented among the group of men who have sex less than once a month, as are those with no relationship at all, the youngest men, those with middle levels of education and men with lower incomes.

Five per cent of the men are not having sex at all at the moment. This is most often linked with youth, single or separated status, and having occasional or no relationships. It's more common among men who have only ever had one partner, and for those who lost their virginity aged 20 or later.

Can't Get No Satisfaction

However, the evidence suggests that most men – and not just those having little or no sex – are not entirely satisfied with their personal sexual status quo. Almost six men out of ten would like to have sex more often. This finding was reflected in the small group discussions, where the young men were particularly likely to say they wanted more sex.

Men across every age group say they would like more sex, but it is a plea most often made by single men and those with occasional relationships or none, rather than men with a regular partner. Seventy-five per cent of the two-timers also feel they'd like more sex than they currently get! In terms of sexual activity, the more frequently a man has sex, the less likely he is to complain he's not getting enough. However, 29 per cent of men having sex four times a week or more would still like more. This compares with 83 per cent of men having sex less than once a month.

Thirty-nine per cent of our men consider that they have about the right amount of sex. A man's contentment with his sex life does not seem to vary consistently according to his age, education, income, type of employment or whether he's a father. Single men are less likely to say their current level of sexual activity is ideal, as are those with occasional or no relationships and two-timers, when compared with men who have a regular partner. Again, there is a direct correlation with activity – the more sex you have, the more likely you are to say it's enough.

Men find the idea of having too much sex a very strange concept; only 1 per cent make this complaint. In the group discussions, the only example of sexual overload was given by a 19 year old man who talked of having too much sex during a relationship with a voracious older woman. This was the only evidence we came across that supports the cartoonist's view of the modern male being forced into action by his rapacious Amazon partner!

Law of Desire

We explored male/female differences in desire for sex in some depth during the group discussions. Most men involved confirmed that they would like to make love more frequently and that it is their partners who restrict how often it occurs. A married 30 year old put it this way, 'I'd never say no, even if she was feeling a bit randy and I wasn't. Whereas the other way round, we wouldn't have it.' A cohabiting 25 year old told a similar story: 'She decides how much, because even if you really want it, if she doesn't – that's it. You could never expect someone to say yes all the time.'

It seemed important for men in the groups to see themselves as constantly ready for sex. More than simply a physical desire, it is a crucial part of their self-image that 'men want it all the time'. A pattern can easily become established in a relationship where the woman dictates how much sex there will be: the man tries his luck and is sometimes accepted, sometimes rejected. If the woman takes the initiative, men will rarely refuse, even if they're not feeling particularly turned on. This may relate to the fact that men are said to be more easily aroused than women.

Some men claimed that women use this in a manipulative way: be a good boy and you'll get your oats. They believed that women are well aware of the power of their sexual attractiveness as well as their power of refusal, but it was something that they accepted cheerfully enough. It's almost as if it suits men in some way to have handed over this power to women, and there are several possible reasons for this tolerance of rejection.

Firstly, it confirms man's self-image as a healthy sexual animal. If women are not always willing to have sex, it's easier for a man to believe that he is permanently hungry for more. He therefore rarely has to face the situation where he doesn't actually want sex, which would threaten his masculinity. It might also be because men are primed to accept refusal from time to time, in deference to menstruation. There's also the acknowledged game in some relationships in which the woman exchanges sex in return for the man taking her out, doing a particularly tedious household chore like decorating, or earning brownie points in another way. Men in our groups reacted in an extremely emotional way to the idea of rape, and were keen to emphasise that they would never dream of forcing the issue: if a woman says no, she means no.

Hormone Overload

Younger men, especially those not in a steady relationship, tended to have a rather different perspective from their elders, and were much more likely to be constantly on the look-out for sex. As one cohabiting 39 year old commented: 'I bet the 57 per cent (who would like more sex) is mainly youngsters. They want it all the time. Their lives are centred around "pulling a bird" – eyes darting round everywhere.' Privacy seemed to be more elusive for younger men and those in a relationship but not living with their partner. This stops them from having as much sex as they would like. Evenings when their parents go out are precious. They say that their partners are just as eager for sex and unlikely to refuse them, though their girlfriends may be less willing to take the risk of being seen or caught. Younger cohabiting men also made the point that they might have enough sex with their girlfriends, but would ideally like to have more sexual partners.

MEN ON SEX

Monogamy is back in style, it would seem, with most men in our survey having been faithful to one partner during the last 12 months. The majority also want more sex than they get: a classic case of demand exceeding supply. And while older men tend to seek quality, for some younger men – like this single 19 year old – the goal is quantity: 'In an ideal world you'd be able to meet someone at a bus-stop, go for a drink, take them home and bonk their brains out – and then go back home to your girlfriend for dinner.'

FIRST RESPONSE PROFILE

Name:	James
Age:	27
Occupation:	Self-employed
Lives:	South East
Education:	'O', 'A' levels, degree
Sexuality:	Heterosexual
Relationship:	None
Virginity loss:	16, didn't enjoy it much
Number of partners:	10

Number of Partners

My relationships have tended to be over long periods. I've had a number of six- to nine-month relationships, then one big two and a half year relationship where I lived with a woman; a few short flings, then a big serious number. After I split up with my long-standing girlfriend, I was celibate for 18 months – it was horrendous. I wondered how long it would be before I became a virgin again. According to a friend, it's seven years!

Sex Within a Relationship

In a long-term relationship, sex goes up and down. After two years, it deteriorated because the relationship was deteriorating. It was steady – probably two to three times a week. But it's different if you're living with someone – the opportunity is there seven days a week. If you're not living together, you might do it twice a week, but several times a night. I was 25 before I understood what my libido was. It goes up and down. It's not like I have to go and find women all the time, but if I am with someone – yes, I get horny.

Keeping Count

The numbers for the younger group are not static. The number would probably have gone up since the survey was done. I'm sure they're faster-moving. You have more girlfriends when you're younger. I never flew through girlfriends, but I think the older you get, the longer the periods are you spend between girlfriends.

It's odd some men can't remember how many partners they've had. I find it perplexing that those without a relationship have forgotten. With the two-timers – is it a guilt thing, and they're trying to put it out of their mind and don't want to admit it to themselves?

As for people having sex once a month – there could be different reasons for that. Is that sex once a month with the same person? If they're in a steady relationship, it's a duff one. Or if they're going from partner to partner, it ties in with the higher number of single people and men in occasional relationships.

Why Aren't People Having Sex?

If people are celibate, it's probably because they're not in a relationship or they could still be virgins. I could think of other examples – they might be religious. I could say I'm celibate at the moment, but not out of choice! To say you're celibate infers a conscious decision not to have sex, rather than not being able to get it with who you want. Celibate doesn't just suggest a famine of sexual encounters!

I think people will want to find out where they slot in – it's a confirmation that you're not abnormal or doing anything stupid.

MEN ON SEX

People read this sort of information on a very personal level. I know where I fit in and I'm quite happy about my sexuality. But there are a lot of people who aren't happy with their sex life. Maybe they don't want sex as much as their girlfriend does, or their sex life has fallen off. They want to know if it's normal for your sex life to deteriorate over time.

Where Do Men Get Their Information about Sex?

A lot of men read women's magazines. They learn about the opposite sex from reading girlfriends' or sisters' copies of *Cosmo*. I've read hundreds of them, and find them more fascinating than porno mags. They tell you more about the opposite sex than pictures of naked women. A lot of men's conversations are ridden with bravado and are maybe a little distorted. It may make men who haven't got the same ability to bullshit feel more concerned about sex. Mostly, you learn by experience, though. Also, a large number of people read books like *The Joy of Sex* and *The Secret Garden*. Anyone would find these riveting reading, unless you're a complete prude.

What Affects the Number of Partners You Have?

For me, I definitely think it's harder to find or meet people now that I like. I've got a lot of friends in stable relationships, and they don't think about it at all. For those not in a relationship, the general consensus is that it's so hard to meet people these days. Maybe it's a London thing, maybe it's a job thing. Personally, I'm fairly picky and I'm not prepared to have sex for the sake of having sex: I want to make love. A friend's just become recently single and he's just knocked off a couple of people. So he has sex for the sake of it. I think it can lead to too much hassle and aggro, and invariably, it isn't completely guilt-free. So I'm relatively happy waiting till I meet the right person. Then I want to have sex like a rabbit to make up for lost time!

5.

The Nitty Gritty

It's time to delve deeper into the sexual habits of British men. To discover exactly what men *do*, we asked about their experiences, ranging from masturbation and foreplay to pornography and anal sex.

HANDS-ON EXPERIENCE

We saw in the last chapter that most men say they would like to have sex more often. This may well explain why almost 40 per cent of our sample masturbate at least once a week and only one man in five says that he never does so. Here are the full results.

HANDS UP!

More than three times a week	13%
One to three times a week	25%
Two or three times a month	15%
Less often	23%
Never	21%
Not stated	3%

Men under 24 are more likely than any other age group to masturbate more than three times a week. The rate doesn't vary

MEN ON SEX

according to whether you are a manager or a clerk, skilled or unskilled, but it does make a difference if you're unemployed. Forty-five per cent of these men (ten respondents) say they masturbate more than three times a week. Single and separated men are much more prone to onanism than those who are married, and having children also seems to have an inhibiting effect on men. Among men with occasional relationships and two-timers, one in five masturbate upwards of three times a week, compared to one in six who have no current partner and just one in 11 of the men with a regular relationship. The highest rate of masturbation, in fact, goes with either having sex a great deal, or very infrequently. It's also linked to having had more partners, losing your virginity early and enjoying that first experience. In other words, it can be either part of a behaviour pattern of high sexuality, or a sex substitute.

One in four men masturbate one to three times a week; again, these are likely to be younger men, particularly in the 25-29 age group. This pattern is linked to higher levels of education, and it's more common for single men and those without children than their married counterparts. One in five of the two-timers and men with regular relationships come into this category, but it's the people with occasional relationships or none at all who have the highest score. This group also includes a higher proportion of men who never have sex.

There's little to distinguish the 15 per cent of men who masturbate two or three times a month, though separated men and those who have sex once or twice a month figure slightly more in this group.

Men who say they *never* masturbate, however, do have recognisable characteristics. It's the youngest men who are least likely to say they never masturbate, while men over 45 are the most likely to make this claim. Abstinence from masturbation is also linked to basic education and earning over £15k. Only 4 per cent of unemployed men say they never masturbate, and while married men and fathers are twice as likely as the rest to fall in this category, men with occasional or no relationships are much less likely than men with partners to say they never do it. Saying you never masturbate is also linked with having fewer partners. Similarly, the more sex you have, the less likely you are to masturbate; those who have very little sex are least likely to say that they never indulge in the habit.

WARMING UP

What do men do to get in the mood for sex? Drinking is a great favourite: for 44 per cent of men, their idea of foreplay is drinking alcohol. Here is a table of all the activities indulged in as part of foreplay during the past year.

THE WARM-UP

Drank alcohol	44%
Watched blue movies	20%
Tied partner up	7%
Used marijuana	7%
Dressed up	6%
Used whips	2%
Took aphrodisiacs	2%
Used coke or crack	1%
Used 'uppers'	1%
None of these	45%

All types of foreplay appeal most to younger men, and least to the over 40s. Married men and those who've only had one partner are very likely to have said none of these activities have played a part in their sexual activity over the last year. The men who lost their virginity later also show a more reserved attitude to warm-up games. However, the men having most sex and the two-timers stand out as foreplay enthusiasts: three-quarters of the men in these groups have indulged in at least one of the preliminaries listed above.

DUTCH COURAGE

Men in the small group discussions did not admit to indulging in any of the more outlandish suggestions on our list, but drinking alcohol was very popular. It was not consciously used as a form of foreplay, but the feeling was that having a few beers could improve sex because it slows down the pace. According to a married 27 year old: 'That's what relaxes me, that slows me down . . . you enjoy it for longer, and she will also be more relaxed because you're giving her more attention.'

MEN ON SEX

Drinking is a young man's game; more than half of the under 24 year olds subscribe to the view that alcohol heightens sexual experience, compared with 37 per cent of the over 40s. Other groups who hit the bottle before they hit the sack include the separated, those with occasional partners and the two-timers. A fondness for alcohol is also more pronounced for men who've had more than five partners and those who have sex more than four times a week – so drinking seems to be an ingredient in the highly sexed personality pattern.

SEX ON SCREEN

Blue movies attract an audience which crosses the categories of age, education, income and types of employment; they are all equally keen. Everyone in the group discussions had seen porn films, but as with drinking, they were not necessarily part of foreplay. Many men associated them more with a jokey, all-male environment. Few reported women being particularly turned on by blue movies, which tended to limit their popularity as a prelude to sex! 'My wife wanted to see one, but she found it more of a turn-off than anything else. It wasn't a turn-off for me, but I do think your imagination's more fun,' said a married 43 year old. Another man described a similar reaction from his wife: 'My other half goes hot and cold on blue movies. Sometimes she doesn't mind if we sit there and we happen to have one. Other times I suggest, "Why don't we get the old film out tonight?", and it's, "No, I don't want to watch that."

Single men are less likely to watch them than married, cohabiting or separated men, while two-timers rate blue movies twice as highly as men with regular, occasional or no relationships. They appeal more to the highly sexed group of men who've had more partners and who have most sex; men who have been faithful to one partner and those having little or no sex are much less concerned with sex on screen.

NO PAIN, NO GAIN

Tying your partner up is three times more common for the young than the old, but holds its appeal across men in all education, income and employment categories. Separated men are more likely to have tied their partner up. This behaviour is also linked in our sample with early, unenjoyable loss of virginity, a finding which confirms the suggestion that sado-masochistic tendencies may originate from an unpleasant first experience of sex. The group of men most likely to 'crack the whip' includes slightly more of those who are separated, two-timers, men earning over £25k and men who have sex more than four times a week.

CHEMICAL HIGH

Smoking marijuana as part of foreplay appeals more to unemployed people, men under 24, those with basic education and men earning less than £15k. It's not a regular indulgence for married men or fathers; unmarried cohabitors, single men and those without children are more likely than others to roll up the wacky baccy before sex. The more partners a man has had and the more sex he has, the more likely it is he smokes marijuana as part of foreplay.

Young, separated and unemployed men are more likely than other groups of men to be among the very small percentage who take aphrodisiacs. So too are the men who have sex more than four times a week: could this be their secret? Only very small numbers take coke or crack, while fans of uppers include men having sex most often and the unemployed.

GETTING DOWN TO IT

We gave men a list of variations on a sexual theme and quizzed them not only on what they'd done, but on what they'd like to do and what they've absolutely no intention of doing. Men in the small discussion groups implied that they might be interested in some of these variations on straight sex, but that they wouldn't dare suggest them as their partners wouldn't consider such practices. The table on the following page illustrates what men have ever done, and what they've experienced in the last year.

Most men in the small group discussions had experienced oral sex with a woman, and pornographic films and magazines. They were extremely keen to find out how many men had had sex with a prostitute – a subject which fascinated them. Having sex with more than one person was assumed to be two women with one man, and this was admitted as a common fantasy. Men also

SEXUAL VARIATIONS	HAVE DONE	DONE LAST YEAR
Had oral sex with a woman	85%	69%
Read a soft porn magazine	81%	41%
Watched a soft-porn film/video	77%	42%
Watched a hard-porn film/video	61%	31%
Read a hard-porn magazine	52%	20%
Watched a live sex show	28%	5%
Used sex aids	24%	13%
Had anal sex with a woman	21%	8%
Had sex with more than one person at a time	10%	2%
Had sex with another watching	9%	2%
Had sex with a prostitute	9%	2%
Practised S & M/bondage	7%	3%
Had oral sex with a man	4%	2%
Had sex (but not full intercourse) with a man	4%	1%
Had anal sex with a man	2%	1%

tended to be more interested in watching other people having sex than in being watched themselves. Some took the attitude that these kind of practices only come into play when ordinary sex becomes boring and needs to be spiced up a bit. This was thought to happen when couples have been together for a while, or when people get older and are keener to explore different sexual activities. 'You may find you need it in 10 or 15 years' time. There are some people who for one reason or another wouldn't experiment with things at a young age, and then they try it, say bondage, at a later age, and find that they like it,' said a married 39 year old.

A married man living in the South West said he hadn't tried any of these activities, and was perturbed by the inference that he was abnormal: 'Having read this questionnaire and thought carefully about each answer, I feel extremely aged, old-fashioned, and that the world and its current experiences have passed me by – yet I'm only 44! Do I have to appraise my sexual activities, as I appear to be "out of step" with everyone else because of the variety of sexual experiences others could be having? What, who, whom is normal?'

Generally, less than half the men who have tried these activities at some time in the past have indulged in them during the last 12 months. The overwhelming exception to this rule is oral sex with a woman; those who've tried it are very likely to have continued to do so. There is a correlation between experience and activity: the more partners you've had and the more sex you're having, the more likely you are to have had oral sex with a woman in the past year.

PORN AGAIN

Reading soft-porn magazines is another activity practised almost universally. They gain least votes from men who've only had one partner, and most from the two-timers. Although four out of five men have read a soft-porn magazine in the past, only two out of five admit to doing so in the last year. These men are likely to have a middle level of education and to be living with a partner but without children. Single men are also more likely than married men to have a stack of girlie mags under the bed. An interesting pattern emerges for the men who have sex less than once a month. Half of these men have read a soft-porn magazine in the last year. They are also more likely than average to have read hard-porn magazines and watched hard- and soft-core films or videos. These findings suggest that men having very little sex use pornography as a substitute.

Young men are more likely to switch on soft-porn films and videos than the older generation: only 66 per cent of the over 40s watch soft-porn films and videos, compared with 81 per cent of the under 24s. Men in their late 20s are particular devotees of porn videos and films in the past year, and also appear to be keener than most on other types of soft and hard porn. Porn films appeal to the two-timers, and their popularity rises with the number of partners a man has had. Men who've had more than ten partners are much more likely to have indulged in porn films or videos than those with only one partner. Half of the cohabitors and more than half the two-timers have seen a soft-core video or film in the last year, but separated men are much less interested in them.

The over 40s are not as keen as younger men on hard-porn films and videos. Fans of hard porn are likely to be two-timers and men living with a partner but without children. Cohabitors prefer hard porn on film or video rather than in print – possibly because watching it on screen can be a joint activity!

STAGE, AIDS AND SODOMY

Just over a quarter of men have been to a live sex show, and they tend to be aged between 25 and 39. The richest men – those earning over £25k – are twice as likely as the low earners to have paid to see sex on stage. Married men and fathers are also keener on live sex shows as are, of course, those prime sex consumers – the two-timers. Men who've had the most partners are most enthusiastic about sex shows, whereas only one in six of the men faithful to one person have ever seen one. Only one man in 20 has been to a live sex show in the past year, and this hardly varies across different ages, or income, education and employment levels. Those least likely to have paid for this kind of entertainment in the last 12 months are those living with children under the age of four and men who've been faithful to one partner.

A quarter of men have used sex aids. Men under 24 are less keen on them, those earning over £25k most. Forty per cent of the cohabitors have used sex aids on occasion, along with more of the two-timers and a higher percentage of fathers than non-fathers. Men in their late 30s are the most enthusiastic users over the past year, whereas the over 40s are much less interested. Men earning over £25k are also likely to have used sex aids recently (money can't buy you love, but it certainly can get you a blow-up doll).

Men in their late 30s are the group most likely to have had anal sex with a woman. Enjoying this practice is linked to basic education and earning over £25k. Cohabitors, separated men and fathers are keener on this activity than married, single men and those without children.

GROUP ACTIVITIES

One man in ten of our sample has had sex with more than one

person at a time. This activity appeals most to men who have the most sex, those earning over £25k and men in higher forms of employment. Troilism is also more popular with cohabitors and separated men than with those who are married or single. One live-in lover from the discussion groups definitely counted this as one of his fantasies: 'Yes, two good-looking women, I wouldn't say no!' but added, 'I wouldn't necessarily want my partner to be one of them.'

Voyeurism holds most appeal for the older men and those with basic education. Cohabitors, separated men and fathers are keener than married or single men, or those without children. None of the men in their late 30s and those with children under the age of nine have indulged in voyeurism or troilism over the past year. Married men also have a low score here. Men who've had ten plus partners enjoy both activities more than the less experienced men, while 6 per cent of men who have sex less than once a month have indulged in troilism in the last year.

PAYING FOR IT

The men who've had sex with a prostitute are most likely to be separated, two-timers and those who've had most partners. The richest men pay for sex more than those with lower incomes. An unexpected finding here is that men without a relationship are most unlikely to have had sex with a prostitute. Although you might imagine men who don't have a partner would be the most likely customers for prostitutes, our results suggest that they prefer substitute activities such as porn films and magazines. Men who've had less than five partners are also less likely to have visited a prostitute.

SLAP AND TICKLE

Rich men enjoy S & M and bondage: those earning over £25k are twice as likely as men earning less to have taken part in sado-masochistic activities. It appeals to all age groups, though slightly less to the youngest men. Men having the most sex and those who've had more partners are more likely to indulge in S & M, whereas those with one partner and men who never have sex take a particularly dim view of it. S & M heads up the group of practices which attracted less than 5 per cent of our men in the last year. In the group discussions, a married 27 year old gave the reason why he wouldn't be getting involved in sado-masochism: 'My wife would definitely not be interested in tying up, whips, black leather stuff, anything. That is just not her scene.'

Since we conducted this survey, sado-masochistic acts between consenting adults in private have, effectively, been banned. Lord Lane's ruling on 19 February 1992 means that 7 per cent of the men in our sample could now be prosecuted for assault. In his view: 'The satisfying of the sado-masochistic libido does not come within the category of good reason.' Men in our small group discussions, however, had a more relaxed approach to the subject, and felt that sado-masochism operated on a sliding scale ranging from harmless to violent activities. 'I can't imagine wanting to receive or inflict pain during the sexual act, but I can accept that there's something rather different about tying someone up to a bed than there is about slapping nine kinds of shit out of them,' said a married 37 year old.

GAY SEX

The least popular activities involve sexual acts with men. This is hardly surprising since only 2 per cent describe themselves as homosexual, with a further 1 per cent saying they are bisexual. Those who've had oral sex with a man tend to be under 24, cohabiting and single rather than married or separated. However, the highly sexed group also scores more highly here: 8 per cent of men with more than ten partners and 9 per cent of those having the most sex say they have had oral sex with a man.

Having sex, rather than full intercourse, with a man appeals most to men with higher education, cohabitors, single men, those with occasional relationships and the two-timers. It seems to be connected to a lot of sexual experience: 9 per cent of the men with more than ten partners claim to have had sex with a man.

The least popular sexual activity for men in our sample is anal sex with a man. It appeals to 7 per cent of cohabitors (six respondents) and 6 per cent of two-timers (two respondents). The figure for married men is just 1 per cent, and it's unknown among the men in our sample who've only had one partner, those who have sex one day a week, and men who never have sex these days.

FAST FORWARD

But what plans do our sample have to expand the range of their sexual activities? We asked them which practices they would like to take part in at some unspecified time in the future; the results are in the following table.

Men in our sample are generally keen to continue their current sexual activities. There are, however, a number of areas where they'd like to turn today's fantasy into tomorrow's reality. Although only 2 per cent of our men have enjoyed troilism or voyeurism in the past year, many more would like to, given the chance. The 'three in a bed' scenario appeals to 31 per cent of the sample, particularly the young men under 24 and those earning up to £15k. Only a quarter of married men and fathers are interested in the idea, compared with 52 per cent of the unemployed and 49 per cent of the two-timers! Men living with children under the age of four and those who've had only one partner have least time for this fantasy. By contrast, two out of five

I'D LIKE TO ...

Have oral sex with a woman	63%
Have sex with more than one person at a time	31%
Watch a soft-porn film/video	30%
Use sex aids	28%
Watch a hard-porn film/video	28%
Read a soft-porn magazine	27%
Go to a live sex show	22%
Read a hard-porn magazine	21%
Have anal sex with a woman	19%
Have sex with another watching	12%
Practise S & M/bondage	10%
Have sex with a prostitute	5%
Have sex (but not full intercourse) with a man	2%
Have oral sex with a man	2%
Have anal sex with a man	1%

MEN ON SEX

men who've had more than ten partners are keen to experience troilism – so too are those who have sex less than once a month.

Voyeurism appeals to all age, income and education groups, but holds a particular fascination for the unemployed. Married men and those who've only had one partner are not keen to have sex with another person watching, though 30 per cent of the two-timers think it's a good idea, as do 22 per cent of men with ten plus partners.

Having anal sex with a woman is something which only 8 per cent have done, but which 19 per cent would like to experience. Young men and the unemployed are more likely to have this on their 'to do' list, as are the cohabitors and men without a relationship. It also appeals to men who've had more than ten partners and those having sex more than four times a week.

Men who have sex less than once a month appear to inhabit a particularly rich fantasy world. They are the most likely to dream of anal sex with a woman, troilism, S & M and sex with a prostitute. They also have a higher than average desire to indulge in voyeurism and use sex aids in the future.

The possibility of using sex aids appeals to 28 per cent of men. They hold more fascination for younger men, cohabitors, men without children and those with occasional relationships. Sex aids also interest men who've had five or more partners and those who have sex more than four times a week. But they appeal most to men who lost their virginity early.

Only 5 per cent of our sample have been to a live sex show in the last year, yet 22 per cent would like to have the opportunity in the future. This appeals to all ages and all levels of income, education and employment. Separated men like this idea, but men without a relationship are less enthusiastic.

Ten per cent of men look forward to a little S & M, compared with the 3 per cent who've tried it in the past year. They tend to be younger men, single and those in occasional relationships. Men who've had five or more partners have a predilection for bondage, whereas it's of less interest to the men who have most sex. Again, we found that unenjoyable loss of virginity is related to a subsequent desire for an element of pain during sex.

A fair percentage of men are keen to continue to watch porn films and videos, and – to a slightly lesser extent – to read hard- and soft-core magazines. Men earning over £25k are the keenest on all these types of pornography, as are the cohabitors and men living with a partner but without children.

Men thinking about the possibility of having sex with a prostitute are more likely to be young, single and with occasional relationships. A significant 12 per cent of men having sex less than once a month would consider going to a prostitute in the future.

The cohabitors are more likely than most to look forward to having some form of sex with a man, as are those who've had more than ten partners.

NO, THANK YOU

The next stage involved men's decisions on what they have absolutely no intention of doing. The table which follows shows their replies.

NO WAY!

Have anal sex with a man	87%
Have oral sex with a man	84%
Have sex (but not full intercourse) with a man	81%
Have sex with a prostitute	63%
Practise S & M/bondage	60%
Have sex with another watching	49%
Have anal sex with a woman	44%
Have sex with more than one person at a time	32%
Use sex aids	26%
Go to a live sex show	24%
Read a hard-porn magazine	19%
Watch a hard-porn film/video	16%
Read a soft-porn magazine	9%
Watch a soft-porn film/video	9%
Have oral sex with a woman	5%

Having sex with a man fills the top three places. However, these figures suggest that although 91 per cent describe themselves as exclusively heterosexual, some of these men are open to

MEN ON SEX

the possibility of homosexual sex. Men in their late 20s are particularly likely to rule out the possibility of homosexual activities, whereas those in their late 30s are more receptive to the suggestion. Men with higher education and those earning between £15k and £25k are also slightly more likely to say sex with another man would be out of the question. Married men are most strongly against oral or anal sex with a man. Those without relationships, however, are more prepared to contemplate both oral and anal sex with a male partner.

A consistent pattern emerges throughout this section: men who've had one partner are much less likely to consider any homosexual activity than those who've had more than ten partners. Men with limited sexual experience and those with a great deal are united in their disapproval of homosexual sex, while men who've only had one partner are strongly opposed to anal sex with a woman, troilism, voyeurism and sex aids. They are also much more likely than their more experienced counterparts to dismiss the idea of S & M, live sex shows and hard-porn films, videos and magazines. Men who lose their virginity late also tend to restrict their sexual practices more than those who start younger. Late starters are particularly likely to say no to oral or anal sex with a woman, troilism, voyeurism, sex aids, sex with a prostitute, live sex shows and all forms of pornography.

Unemployed men are as open as the rest to many of these sexual activities, but show a strong aversion to the idea of visiting a live sex show and to all forms of pornography.

In summary, oral sex with a woman and all forms of pornography come high up the list of practices men have tried and liked, while three-in-a-bed sex has a potent fantasy appeal. These findings confirm that although masturbation may not be the *most* fun a man can have with his clothes off, it's certainly an activity few would oppose. And when two are playing, most men find that alcohol lifts the spirits as part of foreplay, despite the fact that for many of the men in our sample it put a dampener on the occasion when they lost their virginity.

6.

A Bit of What You Fancy

Attraction means different things to different people, and the survival of the species depends on exactly that. If one stereotype did fit all, where would we be? According to Roger Scruton, author of *Sexual Desire*: 'In general, men prefer women who are younger than themselves, lively with regular good looks and not impossibly stupid. Liveliness is vital for sex appeal. It's back to Stone-Age biological programming. Literally, you are attracted by life.'

Within our sample, some definite patterns emerge. One broad definition is that men who are more highly sexed find most physical attributes more attractive than those for whom sex is less of a priority. There are surprises, too. The cleavage – such a potent symbol of sexuality – is much less important to men than mythology, and certainly the tabloids, would have us believe. We'll examine later the specific groups attracted to breasts. Mouths are another example of a universal symbol. Images of lips have been raised to icon status by Warhol's Marilyn pout, and reduced to the mundane as a S.W.A.L.K. on the back of an envelope. Again, they have a specific appeal for certain types of men.

There are also important variations between the men who value psychological attractions over physical attributes, and vice versa. Let's look at the evidence.

WHAT TURNS MEN ON?

The following table shows the overall pattern. We'll examine the

MEN ON SEX

particular appeal of different attributes and regional variations later. For the moment, you may be interested to learn that charm in a woman seems to be particularly important to men in the South, while intelligence is much less important to Northern men.

	THE IDEAL WOMAN	
	1. Good figure	82%
	2. Face	78%
	3. Humour/wit	70%
=	4. Legs	61%
=	4. Eyes	61%
=	6. Breasts	56%
=	6. Bottom	56%
=	6. Intelligence	56%
	9. Dress sense	55%
	10. Charm	53%
	11. Hair	47%
	12. Mouth	36%
	13. Height	16%
	14. Success	9%
	15. Money	7%

We'll look at the possible reasons why success and money are so unattractive later. First, let's go to the top of the list. Body language speaks volumes, according to our men. Four out of five in the sample say a good figure is the main attraction for them. In the group discussions, men agreed that looks are key, and that a woman's figure can initially be more important than her face. However, a woman's face can soon become *more* important. A married 39 year old gives his view: 'Face is important. Sometimes you're walking down the street and you see a lovely looking girl from the back – smashing bum, long blonde hair, looks like the size you like. Turns round and looks as if a bus had hit it. It's very unfortunate.' Hardly how Shakespeare would have put it, but you get the point.

In small group discussions, men suggested that with women they actually meet, physical attractiveness is of fleeting importance – nature's way of getting you interested. They accept that personality factors are more important in the longer term. However, they may find it difficult to distinguish between what they feel and what they *ought* to feel. Some said that their wives did not have ideal looks, but that they had chosen to marry them for other qualities. At the same time, men commented that an attractive wife or girlfriend was something of a status symbol.

One group in particular felt that, in contrast to women, few men were really unattractive. 'Percentage wise, there are a lot more ugly women out there than there are ugly, unattractive men. Most men are more bland. In the female population there are some real beasties,' according to a cohabiting 22 year old. Many women probably hold the opposite view, or would at least temper the statement by saying that an ugly man must have other qualities which compensate for his lack of good looks!

From the physical, we move to the first psychological attribute to appear on the list – humour. The second is intelligence, which takes joint sixth place with breasts and bottom. These may seem strange bedfellows, but it does prove that brains in some way have the same appeal as those well-known companions, tits and bum. Men in the group discussions said that intelligence was attractive up to a point, but only if they felt the woman wasn't cleverer than them. As Roger Scruton said, what's important is an absence of brainlessness, rather than intelligence itself.

Dress sense brought a similar reaction: men mostly only notice its absence. In the words of a single 27 year old, 'Dress sense is like a good sound-track to a film – if it's really good music you don't notice it when you're watching, you just think it's a fantastic film. Somebody should wear clothes they feel good in, and that will speak a lot about them, but you don't necessarily notice the dress sense.' A woman's dress sense is much less important to more educated men than to those whose education stopped at the age of 16.

There is a big drop from the mouth in twelfth position – which 36 per cent of men find a source of sexual attraction – to height (mentioned by only 16 per cent). From the survey, we can deduce that success and money are of limited importance to men, but – as we saw before – money does come quite a long way down men's list of priorities. In the group discussions, some of the men admitted that a woman who had money could be threatening, and therefore less attractive. More of the younger, poorer men ex-

MEN ON SEX

pressed this view, but so did a married 43 year old. 'In some respects, I think a man would feel slightly ill at ease with "success" and "money." I think it comes back to the man liking to feel he's the breadwinner.'

It's interesting to compare the relative powers of attraction that these attributes hold for men of different ages. The following table contrasts the ratings given by men under 24 with those aged 40-45.

	YOUNG MAN'S DREAM	OLDER MAN'S DREAM
Face	84%	74%
Figure	82%	87%
Humour	73%	63%
Intelligence	57%	48%
Dress sense	58%	49%
Eyes	67%	54%
Legs	61%	55%
Bottom	55%	52%
Breasts	51%	63%
Hair	60%	38%

A woman's breasts and a good figure are the only attributes which attract men over 40 more than men under 24. Humour and intelligence also appeal most to men under 35. After that age, men's interest in being amused or mentally stimulated takes a nose-dive. Men aged 30-34 are also more interested in a woman's money than the older generation! In general, young men pay more attention to facial good looks, eyes and height. The youngest group are particularly attracted to hair, which should at least suggest a new angle for shampoo adverts!

Men in their 40s have other priorities, however. They are less likely to want a woman for her money, and don't seem keen to contemplate hair at an age when they're likely to be losing their own. They are also the least interested in legs. What *does* get them going are a good figure and women's breasts.

It's interesting that men over 40 place a higher value on a good figure than they do on a pretty face. It could be that, for an older man, a woman with a 'youthful,' shapely figure is a greater sexual prize for the world to see.

Not surprisingly, those with more qualifications are drawn to intelligent women: only 40 per cent of men with basic education say intelligence is a turn-on, compared with 64 per cent of those with degrees. Men educated to 'A' level standard are particularly keen on psychological attributes – humour, charm and intelligence – but those with the least education are the most avid fans of breasts, bottoms and legs.

This table takes a look at some of the men who find intelligence a turn-on, and some of those who are less attracted by brain power.

INTELLIGENCE ATTRACTS...
64% of men with degrees
40% of men who left school at 16
60% of men aged 30-34
48% of men over 40
64% of managers
46% of men in lower employment
62% of men without kids
50% of fathers
55% of men in regular relationships
36% of two-timers
61% of men who've had five to nine partners
48% of men who've had one partner

Men earning under £15k like a woman who makes them laugh: 73 per cent of these people find humour attractive, compared with 65 per cent of the highest earners. They are also keen on tall women with good legs. The more a man earns, the more likely he is to appreciate successful intelligent women.

As far as employment is concerned, men at management level take much more of an interest in intelligence than those further down the job scale, and these men are also the most attracted by a good figure and a woman's dress sense. Men in higher managerial positions also appreciate height. Out of all these groups, un-

MEN ON SEX

employed people are the most appreciative of a pretty face, humour, eyes and hair. They also show the most interest in the lower half of the body: 69 per cent find bottoms attractive and 70 per cent like legs.

Married men are as keen on a good body as the next man, but are significantly more resistant to the charms of a woman's eyes, hair, mouth and height than the rest. They are also bottom of the league when it comes to appreciating a sense of humour: only 63 per cent of married men find witty women sexually attractive, compared with 76 per cent of single men. So their wives can relax when a tall woman with beautiful eyes starts telling jokes. But they should beware of the woman in a décolleté dress, as breasts are the married man's area of weakness.

Single men, on the other hand, are keen on humour and intelligence, and find money and success alluring attributes in a woman. Eyes, hair and height appeal to them, but breasts and bottoms are lesser attractions.

Men in regular relationships have average tastes: their likes and dislikes run pretty much according to the table of 'The Ideal Woman' on page 56. In comparison, men with occasional relationships put more value on humour: 80 per cent want a woman who can make them laugh. They are also keener on intelligence and a woman who has money! For some reason, men who have occasional relationships seem to focus more on a woman's head than her body: they are particularly attracted to a woman's eyes, hair and mouth, but not that bothered about her breasts, bottom or legs.

Brainpower is most important to men who have no relationship at the moment; breasts and bottoms do not hold much appeal for them. These men are the least interested in a woman's success and the least mercenary. This group is particularly attracted to a good figure, but much less concerned with what a woman is wearing.

A woman's ability to make a man laugh and keep him intellectually stimulated is also important to men who've had between five and nine partners. These men are also the keenest on charm and dress sense. As for matters of the flesh, there's a general pattern: the more sexual partners a man has had, the more he's turned on by women's bodies, and that means everything from her face and body to eyes, hair, mouth, breasts, bottom and legs. In addition, men with a lot of sexual experience are more likely than the rest to go for rich, successful women.

Charm – a quality particularly admired by the two-timers – is also very important to men who have sex more than four times a week: 62 per cent of them are turned on by women who turn on the charm. Eighteen per cent of these highly-sexed men find successful women attractive. Already identified as an ambitious group, they obviously admire the same quality in their women. They like rich women who dress well, and are by far the keenest supporters of legs. The more sex a man has, the more likely he is to be seduced by a woman's hair, mouth and legs.

Men having the most sex are not the biggest breast and bottom fans. That title goes to those who have sex once a week – the Steady Eddies in our survey. They give 66 per cent of their vote to the b'n'b set, in comparison with the average of 56 per cent. Men who lose their virginity late are also particularly attracted to breasts: 62 per cent of late starters find them a turn on, compared to 54 per cent of men who started young. So, whereas popular myth suggests that it's the most voracious men who get a kick out of a woman's breasts, our survey shows they attract a more cautious type who enjoys a moderate, rather than huge, amount of sex.

Men who start their sexual career relatively late are much less interested in a woman's success, money and dress sense, than those who first had sex before they were 16. Nor do late starters have a fascination with women's mouths; only 28 per cent find them sexually appealing, whereas 41 per cent of early learners think mouths are sexy.

Liking a woman to be funny and clever is linked to losing your virginity at an average age, and enjoying it a fair amount, while those most susceptible to charm are likely to have enjoyed their first experience a great deal. If a man enjoys sex the first time, he is also likely to be attracted to breasts and legs.

In the group discussions, men pointed out that different criteria apply according to whether you see someone in a club or in the street, or whether it's someone you've known for a while. A cohabiting 22 year old said, 'If you go to a night club, you'll be looking to pick up something that's good looking. It's rivalry and competition.' On the other hand, according to a married 33 year old: 'If they were on television, you'd tend to look at breast, bottom and legs. But if you were talking to them with a view to the long term, while those things would have caught your eye, it would then be humour and wit.' Many of the men thought that being relaxed in a woman's company was essential to finding them attractive. They seemed to think that while a good pair of legs or a nice bum might grab their attention initially, compatibility proved to be the vital factor.

> MEN ON SEX

Many of the men in our discussion groups also felt that women overestimate the importance of thinness; several men talked of liking curvy women. 'I prefer women to be woman-shaped, to have breasts. I suppose an hour-glass figure is a bit of a naff thing to say, but that shape. Women's magazines perpetuate a myth that women should be anorexically thin,' said a single 27 year old. A further salvo against the slimming business was fired off by a single 30 year old, 'The number of women who've said to me, "God, I must go on a diet – my bum's getting so big, or my thighs", and you look at them and think – what's wrong with them?'

THE NAKED TRUTH

Getting down to the bare essentials, we asked men in our sample whether they found it more sexually appealing to see their partner semi-clothed or stripped to the raw. Here's what they said.

DO YOU PREFER YOUR PARTNER...			
NAKED?	PARTLY-CLOTHED?	IT VARIES	DON'T KNOW
17%	46%	35%	3%

When it comes down to it, men don't necessarily prefer their partner to be naked, and many find a state of undress more of a turn-on. In the small discussion groups, men agreed with these findings, and said that it's more sexy to see someone partly clothed as this whets the appetite, but leaves something to the imagination. 'A bit of trimming's always a bit nice, isn't it?' said a cohabiting 39 year old. A scantily clad woman was felt to add to the air of expectation: 'Again, it is part of the anticipation. Regardless of whether it's a long-standing relationship, it's still part of the build-up to it,' according to a single 30 year old.

These men confirmed the age-old appeal of the stripper, which seems to fulfil a certain fantasy. 'If some woman walked in here completely starkers, that's wonderful. But I'd be more charged up if they came in and started stripping off,' said a married 37 year old.

Men over 40 are the most likely to say they want their partner naked, while it's those in their late 30s who are keenest on seeing them partly clothed. In the groups, a single 19 year old thought it depended on the relationship: 'For me, it varies. If it's a love thing – naked, definitely. Otherwise, partly clothed.' Men in middle management and those who are unemployed are likely to find it sexually appealing when their partner is partly clothed, while men in higher employment tend to say it varies.

Married and single men are equally keen on a partly clothed partner. In one of the groups, a married 32 year old explained that a woman doesn't have to wear fancy lingerie: 'I like underwear, but I don't necessarily like red frilly underwear. In many ways my wife turns me on more with a nice pair of undies on than she does naked. She wears ordinary Marks & Sparks hipsters or whatever, and I think she looks great in them.'

Men in regular relationships are more likely to want to see their partner naked, whereas those in occasional relationships are the keenest on seeing their partner partly clothed. There is little difference according to how many partners a man has had or how much sex he has now. Apart from the men who never have sex these days: many more of these men prefer their partner to be wearing something, and only 8 per cent say it's best if they're stripped off completely.

TAKING CONTROL

A third of men like it when their partner initiates sex, although the majority prefer to take it in turns. We asked men which they found most sexually appealing – making the first move themselves or having a partner who takes the lead. The following table shows their answers.

DO YOU PREFER A PARTNER WHO . . .	
Takes the initiative?	34%
Makes you take the initiative?	4%
It varies	55%
Don't know	7%

These findings show that most men are certainly not looking for a woman who constantly expects a man to make the first move. Men in small group discussions confirmed that although men always like to see themselves as keen for sex, they love it when their partner takes the initiative. As a single 19 year old student said: 'I find it attractive for the woman to take the initiative, because it's a novelty.' It was clear that a woman keen to have sex proves to a man that she's interested and is a confidence boost. However, if the man always has to make the first move, it's difficult for them to know if their partner is enjoying the experience or just 'giving in'. Men found this particular situation both boring and frustrating.

Only 4 per cent of men prefer women who leave it to them to initiate sex. If a man has had more than ten partners, he is more likely to want to take control of the situation. Men who have sex less than once a month have a particularly high score here: 8 per cent like to be in charge, while 12 per cent of separated men prefer to be on top, at least in a psychological sense. One theory which may explain this need for dominance is that these men have an inferiority complex.

Older men are more likely than the young to take the situation as it comes: 60 per cent of men over 40 say their preference varies, compared to only 46 per cent of men under 24. Meanwhile, the youngest men are the most keen on the idea of a woman taking the initiative. However, men with the most education and the highest income are least keen on a woman having her way with them; this may be because they're in control in other areas of their lives and have no intention of losing their grip in the sexual arena. On the other hand, unemployed people are extremely keen for a woman to take them in hand: 48 per cent say they like a partner who takes the initiative. Men without a relationship are in a greater state of confusion than the rest: 16 per cent say they don't know whether or not they like a partner to initiate sex.

ACTIVE OR PASSIVE?

Three out of four men want a partner who joins in the action instead of lying there thinking of England, according to the replies shown in the table opposite.

DO YOU PREFER A PARTNER WHO . . .	
Is active?	76%
Is passive?	1%
It varies	19%
Don't know	4%

The men most keen on having assertive partners tend to be in their late 30s and relatively rich: 82 per cent of men earning more than £25k want women who have an active involvement during sex. Married men – who tend to emerge from our survey as comparatively staid – are surprisingly keen for their wives to be energetic in bed. Eighty-one per cent of them prefer an active partner, in comparison with only 71 per cent of single men. Men who don't have a relationship at the moment are the least sure they want an active partner; only 65 per cent of them find the idea seductive.

In terms of experience and activity, those who are most attracted to the idea of an active partner are men who've had between five and nine partners and those who have sex more than four times a week. It's also linked to a fairly enjoyable loss of virginity.

In the discussion groups, men were very keen on the idea of an active partner. They felt that if one partner is lying there unmoved, both people are left unsatisfied. A single 28 year old pointed out that being passive is open to different interpretations: 'Does "passive" mean just lying there, or just taking more of a passive role and not controlling who does what or when? In which case, passiveness does have its place sometimes.' Some also felt that the response 'it varies' could include times when the man just wanted to have sex. In this case, there could be less foreplay and the whole business would be over quickly, so would involve less obvious participation by the woman. At this point, some of the younger, more liberated types acknowledged that there are also (fairly rare) occasions when women want to have sex rather than 'make love'.

A minuscule 1 per cent of men prefer a woman to take a submissive role during sex. These men who like to dominate are slightly more likely to be those in lower-status jobs, cohabitors and men who've had more than ten partners.

MEN ON SEX A pretty face and a good figure are still the main attractions, while the evidence suggests that very few men are turned on by a woman's success or money. However, men do want women who take an active part in sex, and a third are happy for their partner to take control. The fact that men give intelligence the same rating as a woman's breasts and bottom proves that attraction isn't simply limited to bits that jiggle and wiggle. And men acknowledge that it's personality – not what catches their eye in the street – that's important in the long term.

7.

Sexual Types
(or It Takes All Sorts)

During our analysis of around 500 pages of MORI computer print-out, some definite patterns emerged. Different personalities began to take shape, according to men's sexual activity and type of relationship. Here we identify eight different sexual types: **Sexual Athletes** (men remarkable for either the number of sexual partners they have enjoyed, or the frequency with which they now have sex, and often both); **Two-Timers** (men who are currently cheating on their partner); **Early Learners** (men who lost their virginity before the age of 16); **Live-in Lovers** (men who cohabit outside marriage); **One-Woman Men** (men who remain faithful to their first sexual partner); **Lone Rangers** (men who currently have sex less than once a month – or not at all); **Exes** (men who are currently separated or divorced); and those who have been **sexually abused**. We shall see what attributes men in each of these groups tend to share, and illustrate each category (with the exception of the sexually abused group) by selecting appropriate questionnaires from our sample.

SEXUAL ATHLETES

Twenty-five per cent of the non-virgins in our sample (191 men) have had ten or more sexual partners. Eleven per cent say they have sex at least four times a week, while 2 per cent claim to have it at least daily. There is quite a lot of overlap between these two measures of sexual activity: men who have had more than ten sexual partners are more likely than those with less sexual

MEN ON SEX

experience to have sex every day. However, the two groups have different attributes so we shall examine them separately.

Those who have sex most often are slightly more interested in their careers than those having less sex. They're also interested in money, as are those who have most sexual experience. Both types of Sexual Athlete are highly charged in every sense. Upfront, confident, over-achievers, they see themselves as ambitious, and believe that women are attracted to the kind of man who has his eye on the main chance. They rate themselves as highly sexed, strong-willed and generally in control. The sexually active group believe that women are more interested in how highly sexed men are. Sexual Athletes rate themselves as fun-loving, but not particularly responsible – qualities which they think make women go weak at the knees. They're also convinced they're good-looking, fearless and athletic.

Where behaviour is concerned, almost all men in the most sexually active group have had oral sex with a woman during the past year, and are quite likely to have indulged in voyeurism at some time. They also make more use of prostitutes, and an unusually high percentage of them tie their partner up as part of foreplay. They are keen on most types of pornography, particularly soft- and hard-porn films or videos, and hard-porn magazines. They are also more likely than other men to have had anal sex with a woman during the last year. They anticipate enjoying porn films, videos and magazines, and they are not at all averse to the idea of seeing a live sex show in the future.

Both types of Sexual Athlete are particularly interested in independence and health. Freedom, their homes and their current partners are greatly valued by the most sexually active. People who have had the most partners aren't much involved in leisure activities (perhaps they regard sex as their hobby). However, those who are very sexually active are interested in hobbies. The more sex a man is having, the more likely it is that he'll be indulging in some sporting activity. Sport doesn't seem to be a sex substitute; on the contrary, sexual athletes tend also to be athletes! So it's surprising to find that both measures of a high interest in sex are associated with smoking cigarettes. Smoking marijuana is also considerably higher among those with more than ten partners than among men who've remained faithful to one, and it peaks among the most sexually active. Those who have had the most partners are also slightly more likely to use aphrodisiacs.

Fast food also goes with sexual activity. Men who have sex at least four times a week are most likely to eat fast food. They are also – like the ten-plus-partners group – by far the most likely to have a drink every day of the week. The more partners a man has, the less likely it is that he'll drink less than once a week. Men who have had a lot of sexual partners are particularly likely to endorse the view that men don't do enough to look after their children. They are also much more likely than men who've only had one partner to subscribe to the view that women with children should be allowed to work, and much more likely than the One-Woman Men to support positive discrimination in favour of women. However, men who are very sexually active are strongly opposed to the suggestion that there's too much sex in advertising, nor do they believe that such advertising is demeaning to women. These men feel most masculine in bed, in the pub and at work, and they are the most likely to admire Richard Branson.

Men with a lot of sexual experience are most likely to have experimented with acupuncture. Massage too is at least twice as common among people who have had many sexual partners as it is for any other group. High current sexual activity is also linked with a penchant for massage (while those who currently lead a celibate life are least likely to head for the massage parlour). Those with the most partners and those who are currently most sexually active tend to have lost their virginity early and to say that they are very highly sexed.

But what makes a Sexual Athlete? The tendency to have more than 30 partners is linked with limited education. However, it's also most common among those who are earning more than £25,000 a year, Those with the most partners are also the most enthusiastic masturbators. Masturbation, in fact, goes with either having a great deal of sex or very little, while those who have very little sex are least likely to say that they never indulge in the habit. People who have a lot of sex are likely to fantasise about the person they're with at the time, while those who have had a lot of partners have a particular weakness for Julie Christie (probably a reflection on their age).

With their appetite for sexual experience, Sexual Athletes appreciate the physical aspects of women and are particularly attracted to a beautiful face and a good body. They also identify with the lure of a woman's success and money – the fruits of the ambition they believe they possess themselves. The most sexually active men are particularly interested in a woman's dress sense, mouth and legs. They are also, though to a lesser extent, attracted by hair. Both groups of sexual athletes are breast men.

MEN ON SEX

Men who've had more than ten partners tend to rate their sexual performance as better than average – they're three times more likely to say this than those who have had only one partner. Those who have sex at least four times a week are also much more likely to think that they are better at it, and to believe that they are well-endowed.

Profile of a Sexual Athlete

This single 27 year old man has had between 20 and 30 sexual partners in the past, and between two and four in the past year. He currently has sex four to six times a week. He drinks four to six times a week and goes over doctors' safe drink limits. He lists his priorities (in no particular order) as: a good social life, having a career, job satisfaction, power, freedom, his own home, independence, good male companions, sex and – finally – peace and quiet. He feels men and women have an equally good deal in Britain today, and thinks the balance of power between the sexes is about right.

He has the ambitious, upwardly mobile aspirations that characterise the Sexual Athlete, and thinks women want romantic, fun-loving handsome men who treat them as equals. He considers himself strong, caring and intelligent, as well as highly sexed, fun-loving *and* responsible. In accordance with these last two qualities, he tends to think he would use a condom for sex with a new partner, but doesn't have any opinion on whether he would be put off by a woman who carried condoms, or who was prepared to sleep with him on a first date.

He has taken part in a fairly wide range of sexual practices, and has had oral and anal sex with a woman, experienced troilism and voyeurism, practised S & M, been to a live sex show and enjoyed all types of pornography. In the last year, he's had oral sex with a woman, been to a live sex show and read a soft-porn magazine. He'd like to continue all these practices, but sex with a man or a prostitute is out. He is able to communicate with his partner concerning sex, and feels his sexual performance is a little better than most. He masturbates between one and three times a week and enjoys fantasising.

TWO-TIMERS

A small but distinctive group of the men we contacted believe in having their cake and eating it. Seven per cent of the 473 men currently cohabiting with a woman are cheating on them, either on a regular (3 per cent) or an irregular (4 per cent) basis. As explained in the introduction, when looking at a small group of individuals (28 men), we cannot be certain they are representative of their section of society as a whole. Nevertheless, these men have some interesting characteristics. They have very little time for social life but are extremely interested in money. Independence does not rate highly with them, whereas their health does. They are twice as likely as any other group to consider themselves very fit and much less likely to describe themselves as unfit. They are great sports enthusiasts. Smoking does not appeal to them, nor do they eat much fast food. They do, however, drink more than other groups and it is very unusual to find a Two-Timer who drinks very little.

So far as attitudes are concerned, very few of them subscribe to the view that women get a good deal in Britain today, though they are most likely to endorse the view that the balance of power is too much in women's favour. They disagree with the view that there should be more positive discrimination in favour of women, and none of them would want to have a woman as their boss. To complete their generally chauvinist view of the world, the Two-Timers think it's nonsense to suggest that women are demeaned by advertising.

Like other men, Two-Timers feel at their most masculine at work and during sport. But they are much less likely to say they feel masculine when driving or socialising with a partner, and only 7 per cent feel masculine in a pub. Their heroes include Lord Hanson, Alan Sugar and Nigel Mansell. Almost nine out of ten of this group say they are either fairly or very highly sexed, and none of them has any experience of psychotherapy or psychoanalysis!

Not surprisingly, Two-Timers are well represented in the most sexually active groups. They are the least likely to have had between one and four partners and the most likely to have had more than 30. The Two-Timers are a law unto themselves. In their experience, women don't want strong men. Nor do they think that women are much interested in sensitivity (which is just as well, since they don't consider themselves sensitive). And they don't consider themselves particularly caring or intelligent. In their experience, too, women are not turned on by a man's brainpower, rather by how highly sexed he is. They don't rate themselves as very romantic, though they do fancy themselves as athletes. To their frustration, however, the women they have encountered have not been turned on by athleticism. Nor do they think that women are attracted to an artistic spirit or towards men who treat them as equals. Less expectedly, Two-Timers don't believe that women are after passion, sensuality or tenderness, let alone romance. Instead, they think women want understanding, though they are uneasily aware that this, too, is a dimension on which they don't score highly.

Two-thirds of the Two-Timers think women like men who are fun-loving, but don't believe they value a sense of responsibility. And these men – who want to have their cake and eat it – don't think women want a man who's strong-willed!

These men know what women like, and it's certainly not a man who gives in! None of the Two-Timers believes submission appeals to women: on the contrary, they are the most likely to say men who have the upper hand get a woman going. They think stamina's important, but energy less so. Three per cent have no idea what women want in bed and a further 3 per cent don't care!

Most men in our sample enjoy a blue movie, but the Two-Timers are twice as likely as any other group to use them as part of their foreplay. They are also quite interested in prostitution, sex with two women and all forms of pornography, while they are three times as likely as the rest to have indulged in voyeurism, and to have practised S & M or bondage. Almost all the two-timing men have enjoyed oral sex with a woman in the past year, and they're twice as likely as any other group to have enjoyed anal sex with a woman. Two in five of the Two-Timers have experience of the joys of a gleesome threesome, and more of them have seen live sex shows than men in other categories. They also tend to be hard-porn magazine devotees, but are strongly opposed to the idea of anal sex with a man.

Two-Timers are fantasists. They are much more likely than any other group to fantasise while they're actually having sex and are also prone to give their imaginations free rein while in the bath or in the shower. Half of them fantasise about sex with someone who's not with them, but they are also much more likely than other groups to fantasise about someone they're with at the time. They never fantasise about 'no-one in particular' and are attracted to Felicity Kendal and Gabriella Sabatini – but not Nastassia Kinski. They're much less likely than other men to think about sex when driving or watching films or television. And only

18 per cent are prone to combining socialising with fantasy. But what they *do* love is thinking dirty on the phone. A man just can't be in two places at once, but 26 per cent of Two-Timers find the telephone a useful way to bridge the gap.

From some of the descriptions above, you might assume that Two-Timers are heat-seeking missiles whose systems would go into red-alert at the merest sight of a woman's body. However, the evidence presents a slightly different picture. They are less interested than other men in a pretty face, and only 56 per cent of them are turned on by a good figure, which comes at the top of everyone else's list of attractions. They are left relatively unaffected by a woman's dress sense and eyes, and are almost completely indifferent to her hair. They are also unimpressed by humour and intelligence – a worry, perhaps, about women who might read their game or, worse still, be amused by their antics. Two-Timers, again, are the least interested of all in height, legs, breasts and bottoms. Whereas breasts and bottoms tie with 56 per cent in the overall league table of attractions, two-timing men award them just 39 per cent each.

So what does excite these men? In short, success, mouths and charm. Half of the two-timing men say a woman's mouth can make her sexually attractive, and 61 per cent find charming women seductive.

Two-Timers are by far the most likely to be tempted by a naked partner: 41 per cent of them like to see their partner stripped, compared with only 17 per cent of the whole sample. They are the most keen to have a partner who is active during sex: 86 per cent of these men are happy to let the woman make an active contribution, in comparison with the average 76 per cent, and they definitely don't want a passive partner.

Two-Timers have no doubts about their ability to tell their partners what they want or to sense a woman's requirements. They are also the most likely to describe themselves as well-endowed, though the least likely to say that size is important to women. They rate their performance as a lot better than average, and are particularly interested in giving as well as receiving pleasure. This may be a reflection of the fact that two-timing men are the most likely to say that they learned their sexual technique from their own sexual partners.

Profile of a Two-Timer

This married man in his late 30s is having a relationship with a woman who is either married or living with someone else. As with others in his group, he does not list a good social life as a priority, but does value job satisfaction, money, his children and car. Health is also listed as a concern, despite the fact that he drinks every day and consumes more than 35 units a week. He has had more than 30 partners in the past, and between five and nine in the last year. He currently has sex two to three times a week, and masturbates infrequently. Not a fan of condoms, he tends to think he wouldn't use a condom for sex with a new partner. But he wouldn't be put off by a woman who carried condoms, any more than he would lose respect for a woman who wanted to have sex on a first date!

Rating himself as fairly highly sexed, he has experienced fewer sexual activities than some of the other two-timing men. He's had oral sex with a woman, watched a hard-porn film and read a soft-porn magazine, but of these, he has only had oral sex with a woman during the last twelve months.

He rates himself as fun-loving, and thinks women want men who are caring, sensitive, fun-loving, romantic and understanding. In bed, he believes women's major needs are for affection and stamina. His needs in bed are a partner who is naked, active and takes the initiative, and he's attracted by humour and a woman's breasts.

This man does not share the chauvinistic tendencies of other Two-Timers: he says men get the best deal in Britain, but that they have too great a share of the power. Definitely in favour of women with young children going out to work, he strongly supports positive discrimination in favour of women.

EARLY LEARNERS

Twenty per cent of our sample (161 men) lost their virginity below the age of legal consent (16). It's interesting to compare these men with those who entered the sexual lists unusually late (after the age of 20) or Mr Average (the 54 per cent of the sample who had their first sexual experience between the ages of 16 and 19). The Early Learners set great store by a good social life and are significantly more interested in money and freedom. Early Learners rate themselves fitter than those who came to sex late and they're less likely to consider themselves overweight. However, those who lost their virginity early are four times more likely to be smokers than those who lost it late – suggesting a pattern of people who are impulsive in more ways than one. In keeping with this, the Early Learners are fast-food enthusiasts.

The quality of first sexual experience also seems to be important. Those who didn't much enjoy losing their virginity are very interested in their partners. Early Learners and those who enjoyed the experience tend to become heavier drinkers (while Late Starters are the most likely to drink very little. The tendency to be abstemious with drink is also associated with joyless loss of virginity, perhaps indicating a personality uncomfortable with pleasure.) The heaviest drinkers in our sample are certainly those who lost their virginity early and enjoyed the experience. Early Learners and those who enjoyed it say they feel most masculine when in bed, at work, while driving or on holiday. They are also much more likely to feel masculine when out socialising with their partner than those who lost their virginity later. Those who didn't enjoy the experience first time are most likely to say they feel masculine during sport.

Early Learners are more likely to entrust themselves to the psychotherapist's couch than those who lost their virginity after the age of 20. In contrast, the Late Starters take their problems to a more conventional source: they are three times more interested in religion than their early starting colleagues.

Early loss of virginity is a strong predictor of later sexual behaviour. The Early Learners are more likely than the rest to have sex every day and to have had more than 30 sexual partners. The practice of tying a partner up as part of foreplay, interestingly, is associated with the early and joyless loss of virginity. Early Learners tend to be more confident that they can make their desires known to their partners, whereas those who didn't enjoy their introduction to sex are most likely to say that they can't express what they want. Early Learners are also more confident that they know what their partner wants and to have learned their sexual technique from partners.

From the evidence in our survey, men who lose their virginity early are upbeat, upfront optimists. Strong, ambitious and upwardly mobile, they consider themselves highly sexed, fun-loving, handsome and confident. They are not afraid of being labelled money-orientated, and come across as less caring, shy and understanding than the men who leave it longer before embarking on their sexual careers. They are also less likely to think they're intelligent than men who lose their virginity later.

They do, however, think they possess one quality usually

associated with the more retiring sexual types – being artistic. To complete their self-assessment, they also tend to be comparatively more romantic, fearless and athletic – all essential for the men who literally leapt into bed at the first opportunity.

Asked to say what women want in a man, Early Learners describe themselves! In their view, women like a man on the make who's sure of himself, loves sex and being in control. These men are less likely to believe that being sensitive, intelligent and responsible is the way to a woman's heart.

Enjoying blue movies as part of foreplay is a predilection linked to early loss of virginity, as is smoking marijuana. Early Learners tend to believe women want passion in bed, and have more faith in the attraction of a man who is dominant, and has stamina and energy.

These men tend to get involved in a wide range of sexual activities. In the past year, they are extremely likely to have had oral sex and more likely than most to have had anal sex with a woman, read hard-core porn magazines, used sex aids and gone to a live sex show. Men who lose their virginity before the age of 16 are also more likely than those who started later to have experienced troilism and to have had sex with a prostitute.

The earlier a man loses his virginity, the more he's turned on by a woman's dress sense, success and money: physical and social impact count for the Early Learners. They are also more likely than Late Starters to prefer a partner who takes the initiative. Early Learners and those who enjoyed their first experience of sex are more likely than average to fantasise about someone they're with at the time and to let their thoughts drift towards sex at a party or in the pub. At work, while travelling and on the phone are also favourite fantasy times for these men. However, they are much less likely to fantasise in bed than those whose sexual initiation came later. Early Learners are the most keen on the idea of a woman who would sleep with them on a first date: 36 per cent say they'd still respect her, compared with only 26 per cent of Late Starters.

Profile of an Early Learner

Now aged 19, this Early Learner started his sexual career aged 14-15, has sex four to six times a week and rarely masturbates. He's very confident of his ability to communicate about sex with his partner, and believes it's important for both partners to have equal satisfaction from sex.

He always carries condoms, and would never have sex with a new partner without using one. Equally, he definitely wouldn't be put off if a woman carried condoms, but would lose respect if she was prepared to sleep with him on the first date. He's had between two and four sexual partners in the past, but just one during the last twelve months. He's tried oral sex with a woman and has experience of soft porn, but anticipates taking part in troilism and voyeurism in the future. He's not at all interested, however, in sex with a man, S & M, sex aids, sex with a prostitute or hard porn. Describing himself as sensitive and ambitious, fun-loving and responsible, the only attractions he feels he lacks are good looks, strength, shyness and athleticism.

Most female attributes attract him, with the exception of a woman's money. He believes men get the best deal in Britain today and that the balance of power is too much in favour of men. His 'feminist' views include the ideas that women with children should work, men don't do enough for their children, and that sex in advertising is demeaning to women.

LIVE-IN LOVERS

The 10 per cent of our sample who cohabit outside marriage tend to be career men: they are among the keenest on having a job. They are interested in money, and express a high interest in their partner. Eleven per cent of these men are also quite keen on marijuana. They feel most masculine during sport, and are among the men most likely to feel masculine while gardening or engaging in DIY! A quarter of them also feel manly behind the wheel, socialising with their partner and in the pub.

The cohabitors are very active sexually: they are the men most likely to have sex four to six times a week or more often, and go in for a wide variety of sexual practices. They are more likely than most to have had anal sex with a woman, to have experienced troilism and voyeurism, used sex aids and practised S & M. Pornography tends to appeal to these men. Seven per cent of the cohabitors have had oral or anal sex with a man: as only 6 per cent of cohabitors describe themselves as homosexual, this leaves 1 per cent of 'floating voters'.

Live-in Lovers think women want a man who is understanding, and fun-loving yet responsible. They also rate themselves as more fun-loving and less responsible than the average man. They don't rate being caring or intelligent as highly as their married counterparts. Seventeen per cent of them believe that being highly sexed counts in a man's favour, and 32 per cent rate themselves as such.

The cohabitors rate themselves as more ambitious than average, and one in five says he's upwardly mobile and eight per cent of Live-in Lovers say they're macho, compared with 3 per cent of the whole sample. More of them think they're good-looking, strong-willed and in control than married, single or separated men, but they are less romantic than average, although three-quarters of them believe that this is what women want.

Three-quarters of the Live-in Lovers believe women want affection in bed, followed by tenderness, sensuality and passion. They are also the group most convinced of the power of dominance: 24 per cent of them say women like a man who takes control in bed, compared with only 12 per cent of married men. They rate stamina much more highly than the rest: 40 per cent say staying power counts for a lot, whereas just 22 per cent of those who are married think women want stamina. They also rate energy as important. All in all, the Live-in Lovers think women place a high value on a man who's powerful in bed. Accordingly, 6 per cent of these men (5 respondents) say they like a woman to be passive during sex, which is slightly higher than the average 1 per cent of men who give this reply.

A successful woman can be particularly seductive to Live-in Lovers: 16 per cent of cohabitors say they find success attractive, compared to only 7 per cent of married men. They are the least keen on breasts, but seem to have more interest in women's bottoms than any other group in our sample.

Cohabitors are much less inclined to fantasy than their single counterparts. But when their thoughts do drift towards sex with someone they haven't slept with, it's likely to be when they're lying in bed, out socialising at a party or in a pub. They're also pretty keen on fantasising while watching television or a film. They have a relatively low capacity to be 'mentally unfaithful' to their partners. They are less likely than married or separated men to say they *sometimes* think of someone else during sex, and not one of them says he *always* fantasises about another person when having sex with his partner. Live-in Lovers are more likely than the rest to fantasise about the person who's with them, or about sports personalities. However, a third of cohabitors cannot think of anyone in particular to start up their fantasies.

Profile of a Live-in Lover

A 34 year old man cohabiting with his partner, this man is interested in a good social life, freedom, children, independence, politics, sex, his friends, his car and holidays. He doesn't, however, include his partner on this list of priorities. He has the typical sexual profile of the cohabitors in our survey. Having lost his virginity early (before the age of 14), he now has sex at least once a day, and believes he has about the right amount. Describing himself as very highly sexed, he masturbates between one and three times a week, is fairly confident about sexual communication, and thinks his performance is better than most.

As far as foreplay is concerned, he has tried alcohol, uppers and marijuana. He has also tried absolutely every sexual variation on our list in the past, from oral and anal sex with a man and a woman, to S & M, troilism, voyeurism etc. But during the last 12 months, he has restricted his sexual variations to oral sex with a woman, and he doesn't want to have any homosexual experiences in the future.

In his view, his partner's satisfaction is paramount and he likes a partner who takes the initiative. He thinks he's well-endowed, and that it matters. This Live-in Lover tends to think he wouldn't have sex with a new woman without using a condom. As far as allocating professions to gender, he wouldn't prefer a male lawyer, doctor, surgeon, MP, train or bus driver. Nor does it bother him whether his boss is male or female – but he *would* prefer a female best friend. He is among the few men who admire Jeremy Paxman and fancy Anita Roddick.

ONE-WOMAN MEN

Eighteen per cent of our sample (133 men) have remained faithful to their first sexual partner. What distinguishes these men from their more promiscuous colleagues? They are not particularly interested in a good social life, nor is a career so important to them. They don't rate freedom highly and their drinking habits are the most modest in our sample.

Men who've been faithful to one partner are not generally prone to untamed passions, boisterous behaviour or wildly irresponsible urges. Compared to more experienced men in the survey, they rate themselves the least fun-loving. And, to the best of their knowledge, this is what women want. They are also most reluctant to believe women are eager for men with sex on the brain; and only 17 per cent say they're highly-sexed, in contrast with 38 per cent of men with ten plus partners.

One-Woman Men are more likely than average to think women want sensitive men who're in control; however, they themselves do not feel in control. They don't think it's an advantage to be highly sexed, upwardly mobile or money orientated. In accordance with this 'New Man' profile, they rate themselves among the most caring and sensitive of our sample, and the least ambitious. But they don't feel they have great reserves of willpower, strength and control. This crisis of self-belief is compounded as 64 per cent of them think women go for handsome men, yet only 19 per cent think they're good-looking. Nor do they rate themselves as particularly athletic or romantic, and they suffer from shyness more than more experienced men.

When asked what they like in a woman, less than half say they're interested in charm or intelligence. They're also less concerned than the rest with a woman's dress sense, success or money. When it comes to sex, they are the only group somewhat less in favour of having oral sex with women in the future, and they're least tempted by hard-porn films or videos. Asked what they think women want in bed, they opt for tenderness and affection rather than sensuality or passion.

Of course, none of the One-Woman Men have ever found themselves three in a bed, which is in contrast to 26 per cent of men who've had more than ten partners. But 18 per cent do find the idea of troilism particularly attractive. Hard-core porn magazines hold little appeal for them, however, and only 2 per cent have indulged in voyeurism, compared with 21 per cent of men who've broken the ten-partner barrier. To complete their restrained sexual profile, only 1 per cent of One-Woman Men have ever tried S & M, and none of them has done so during the past 12 months.

What these men *are* interested in is home, partner and religion. One-Woman Men are less likely than those with more experience to feel masculine in bed, while driving, socialising or taking exercise, but more likely to feel manly at home and with their children. They're also fairly conservative when it comes to social attitudes. For example, they are the most likely to say that the balance of power is now tipped too much in favour of women and that women with young children shouldn't work. They are also the least likely to describe women colleagues as friends. For these men, it's important to keep boundaries between their sexual partner and other women, and they think it's vital to have a male best friend.

The One-Woman Men tend not to be rich. Seven out of eight men who earn more than £25,000 a year have had more than one sexual partner. One-Woman Men are also inclined to be shy – more than twice as shy as men who have had more than ten sexual partners.

One-Woman Men restrict their thoughts to their partner to a far greater degree than the rest. Only 12 per cent say they fantasise about someone else when they're having sex with their partner, compared to the average 22 per cent of our men. They are less likely than men with more experience to fantasise during meetings at work, while having a bath or on the phone. A third of One-Woman Men fantasise about no-one in particular. However, 7 per cent of men who've been faithful to one partner also fantasise about a relative.

Profile of a One-Woman Man

This married 26 year old expresses many characteristics typical of the One-Woman Man in our sample. His wife is his only sexual partner, and comments on his questionnaire confirm that monogamy is his ideal. He describes himself as fairly fit, takes part in sport and is an abstemious drinker.

He lists three priorities: his partner, his parents and job satisfaction. He lost his virginity aged 25 or 26, and enjoyed that first experience a great deal. He has sex at least once a day, never masturbates, and thinks he has the right amount of sex. Very confident of communication between himself and his partner, he thinks her satisfaction is more important than his own. He never has sexual fantasies about someone he hasn't slept with.

In terms of sexual experience, the only variation on a theme he has tried is oral sex with a woman, and he definitely does not want to try any of the other practices on our list. He strongly disagrees with the idea that there are women at work he finds attractive, but he does have female friends at work. He tends to think women with young children should work rather than stay at home, and that men don't get enough time with their children. However, he is strongly against positive discrimination in favour of women.

In line with the general characteristics of the One-Woman Man in our sample, he rates himself as caring, sensitive and responsible. However, he goes against the standard type by describing himself as an ambitious, fun-loving, self-confident person who's in control.

LONE RANGERS

Eighteen per cent of the non-virgins in our sample (131 men) say they have sex either less than once a month (13 per cent) or – currently – never (5 per cent). What distinguishes these men? They tend to be very concerned with job satisfaction and the concept of freedom. They rate themselves as unusually fit. They are much less likely to describe themselves as overweight; indeed a significant number of them say that they are underweight. Men who are having sex less than once a month are only a third as likely to be on a diet as the rest of the sample. They are also the least likely to be drinking every day. Drinking very little is particularly common for those who have no current relationship.

Not everyone wants to have sex, and a few men took issue with what they saw as our presumption that there's something wrong with men who are currently celibate. A few expressed the opinion that they don't believe in sex before marriage, and a single 26 year old made the following comment: 'I got the impression that an implicit assumption had been made that regular, or at least occasional, sex is the norm, and that anyone not conforming to that norm has some sort of problem.'

Those 38 men who never have sex currently tend to rate themselves as particularly sensitive, caring and responsible. Fifty-three per cent describe themselves as shy, compared with only 17 per cent of those who have sex more than four times a week. Other factors which may hinder their search for a partner are that 80 per cent don't consider themselves very good-looking and 72 per cent are lacking in confidence. They also lack determination, rating themselves among the least strong-willed and in control.

However, they do consider themselves romantic, understanding and fun-loving. They don't share the ambitious, athletic qualities of the Sexual Athletes, and only 16 per cent say they're highly sexed.

In their opinion, women want men who are handsome, caring, romantic and sensitive. Men who never have sex are less likely to think women prefer men who treat them as equals. Men who have sex less than once a month are more likely than the rest to say women rate stamina very highly, but are less likely than the more sexually active to think women are interested in affection in bed.

On the question of what makes someone sexually attractive to the Lone Rangers, there are important differences between men who have sex less than once a month, and those who currently don't have sex.

Men who have very little sex are among the most drawn to wit: 80 per cent of them are attracted by a sense of humour. Intelligence appeals to them more than to other men, and they are the most likely to be affected by someone's eyes.

Those who are sexually inactive rate humour and intelligence fairly highly, but are the least likely to be taken in by charm. And not one of them would describe success as an attractive feature. They are most concerned with a woman's face and figure, and find eyes sexually appealing. However, only 39 per cent say that clothes can attract their attention; compared with the average 55 per cent of men who find a woman's dress sense appealing, these men are not at all concerned with such physical trappings! Overall, fifty-six per cent of men in our survey are attracted to breasts and bottoms, whereas only 36 per cent of men who never have sex find breasts sexually stimulating. They also find bottoms less appealing than do men who have sex more often.

Men who are currently sexually inactive do not feel masculine during sport. They are very unlikely to admire Richard Branson, Mick Jagger and Gary Lineker. By contrast, Prince Charles draws his fans almost exclusively from men who never have sex! This group almost never indulges in massage, although they are significantly more interested than other men in yoga. Like the One-Woman Men, people who are not currently sexually active are unusually interested in religion.

The Lone Rangers are the most frequent masturbators and fantasists of our sample. The men who have little or no sex fantasise the most, and men who have sex less than once a month have sex on their mind more frequently than those who are sexually inactive at the moment. Just over a third of men in both groups are very likely to think of sex at work, while travelling, and when socialising. Lying in bed is their favourite place to fantasise, and those having sex less than once a month are more keen than most to drift off in the bathroom, or while talking on the phone.

Men having the least sex are more likely than those having more sex to choose someone who is a more distant, unattainable figure as the object of their fantasy. Forty-six per cent of men who never have sex fantasise about someone they know vaguely, compared with only 26 per cent of men having sex more than four times a week. Men who have sex less than once a month are among the most likely of all groups to fantasise about someone who's not with them at the time, one of their friends, someone at work, or someone they've seen once or twice. This is the only group of men to whom Joan Collins seems to hold any appeal. She and Prince Charles may be considered an unlikely pair. The currently celibate are also powerfully drawn towards Nastassia Kinski.

Men who have very little or no sex are generally likely to feel masculine while driving and when in a pub. And those who have sex less than once a month feel particularly masculine during sport or physical exercise. But men who never have sex do not feel masculine when they're at home: only 3 per cent claim this, compared with 19 per cent of men having sex at least four times a week.

Soft-porn films and videos are widely used among people having no sex at the moment; hard porn is also very popular. The frustration experienced by men who have sex less than once a month may explain the finding that they are particularly willing to contemplate anal sex with a woman, troilism or S & M – at some point in the future.

Profile of a Lone Ranger

A single 23 year old virgin, this man places particular value on his social life, job, career, money, freedom, independence and leisure. He masturbates between two and three times a month, doesn't know if he's highly sexed and doesn't care what women want in bed. He fantasises when lying in bed, either about someone not with him or someone he knows vaguely.

He would never have sex with a new partner without using a condom, and wouldn't be put off by a woman who carried them or who'd be prepared to sleep with him on a first date. He's attracted by humour, charm, intelligence, a pretty face, a good figure, and a woman's eyes and mouth. In his view, women want handsome, self-confident men, but he does not rate himself as this type. However, he does think he's caring, intelligent, sensitive, fun-loving, responsible, upwardly mobile, romantic, shy, strong-willed, understanding and after equality. In Britain today, he believes men have the better deal, and that the balance of power is too much in favour of men. He has no preference for a man or woman in the list of professions in our survey.

EXES

Five per cent of our sample (45 men) are currently separated (2 per cent), divorced (3 per cent) or widowed (less than 1 per cent, just four men). A third of these men have a regular partner, and just over a third have occasional partners. Although very interested in job satisfaction, these men do not attribute anything like as much importance to having a career. They are much more interested in freedom than people who are married or cohabiting, and are the most drawn to the notion of having their own home. When it comes to fitness and weight, Exes seem to attach themselves to one of two extremes – they are either very happy or very dissatisfied with their current state. They smoke and drink far more heavily than married men. Heavy drinking (i.e. more than 35 units a week) is twice as common among this group as any other, and they are by far the most likely to drink every day.

They are also twice as likely as any other group to claim that women get the better deal in Britain these days. In keeping with this view that women have a social advantage over men, they are the least likely to say the balance of power is too much in favour of men and significantly more likely to deny that sexual harassment is a problem at work. Most feel most masculine in bed, but only a quarter feel masculine at work. They find a partly clothed partner particularly sexually appealing, and 12 per cent of them say they like a partner who makes them take the initiative in sex. Unsurprisingly, the Exes make most use of marriage counselling. They are three times more likely than men in other groups to turn to psychotherapy or psychoanalysis.

Only one in five describe themselves as being in control, but most do think they're understanding, caring and sensitive. They believe women want men who are understanding and caring, but don't think they put as much value on good looks. They are also more likely than average to think a man exerts a more powerful attraction for women if he's macho, upwardly mobile and money orientated. However, they rate themselves less interested than other groups in ambition, money and social climbing.

Eighteen per cent do, however, think women go for highly sexed men, and they are the group most likely to say they possess this quality. And nine out of ten separated men say women are attracted to fun-loving men, although only six in ten say they know how to live it up.

Separated men are more likely than other marital groups to say tenderness is the quality women want most from men in bed.

MEN ON SEX

They rate sensuality slightly more highly than other men, and also attach importance to affection and passion. A third of these men believe men who can demonstrate stamina are attractive to women. However, they place less importance on being very energetic in bed.

Humour and intelligence are important to separated men: they rate them more highly than do either single or married men. They are also keen on a good figure and a pretty face, but are not particularly drawn to a woman's money or success. Exes are leg men: 71 per cent of separated men say they are captivated by leggy ladies.

Separated men have their own special fantasy profile. They're not that keen on fantasising on the way to work, but many more think about sex if they're travelling to some other destination. In the bath or shower and in front of a TV or cinema screen are favourite fantasy locations for separated men, and 79 per cent of them let fantasy take control when they're lying in bed. Forty-seven per cent of Exes fantasise about someone they know vaguely, and 27 per cent get turned on thinking about someone they've only met once or twice.

Separated men are unusually likely to have had more than 30 sexual partners. They are unlikely to describe themselves as being in control and believe that women want men who are understanding – but not affectionate! They tend to consider themselves well-endowed and are twice as likely as men in other groups to use prostitutes. They are particularly likely to admit that they find it difficult to tell their partners what they want during sex. When it comes to what their partner wants, they again divide into two extremes. Both the 'not very confident' and 'confident' reply are unusually common in this group. Surprisingly, Exes are much more likely to say that their sexual performance is a good deal better than average than men in other groups. However, they are also particularly likely to hold the belief that their own pleasure during sex is more important that that of their partners!

Profile of an Ex

This separated man in his late 20s has several characteristics typical of the Exes in our sample. Fairly fit, he exercises, smokes, and drinks between 22-28 units two to three times a week. Describing himself as fairly highly sexed, he has sex four to six times a week and masturbates one to three times a week. He's had between two and four partners in the past. He's very confident of his ability to communicate about sex, and says his performance is average.

He has experienced oral and anal sex with a woman, troilism, voyeurism, S & M, used sex aids and visited a live sex show. However, he rules out homosexual sex and having sex with a prostitute as possibilities in the future.

In line with other Exes, he believes women have the best deal in Britain today. He tends to think that women with pre-school-age children should go out to work, and that men don't do enough to look after their children. He believes women want men who are both strong and sensitive, fun-loving and responsible, romantic and shy. He also thinks they like men with sex and money on their minds!

THE SEXUALLY ABUSED

Sexual abuse of children is a dark subject that is increasingly coming out into the open. As more children are encouraged to report cases of abuse, the numbers of people affected have to be continually revised. Recent estimates stand as high as 10 per cent of children. The NSPCC estimates that 5,400 children in the UK were sexually abused in 1990 – which represents a great increase since the early 80s. But these are conservative figures, based on *reported* cases of abuse, which are necessarily much lower than the real number. Their figures also include fewer older children, as they are much less likely to be reported by outsiders, or to admit to the abuse themselves.

We asked the men in our sample if they had been subject to sexual abuse in childhood, giving the following definition: 'A child (anyone under 16 years) is sexually abused when another person, who is sexually mature, involves the child in any activity which the other person expects to lead to their own sexual arousal. This might involve intercourse, touching, exposure of the sexual organs, showing pornographic material or talking about sexual things in an erotic way.'

Six per cent of the men in our survey say that they were sexually abused as children. Of these 48 men, 37 were willing to answer questions about the experience. Our figures show that sexual abuse of children is twice as common in the South as in the North or Midlands, although the numbers involved are too small to constitute a reliable trend. There is a high incidence of child

MEN ON SEX | abuse among the high earners, the unemployed, separated men, those with ten or more partners, and people who did not enjoy losing their virginity.

HOW OFTEN DID IT HAPPEN?

Once	44%
More than once with the same person	29%
With two different people on separate occasions	8%
With three or more different people on separate occasions	19%

Abuse peaks at the ages of seven and 13. When the abuse occurred, 4 per cent of children were aged six or less; 20 per cent aged seven; 5 per cent aged eight; 6 per cent aged nine; 13 per cent aged ten; 3 per cent aged 11; 15 per cent aged 12; 26 per cent aged 13; 6 per cent aged 14; and 2 per cent aged 15. These figures tie in to some extent with NSPCC figures for 1990, where boys are over-represented in the five- to nine-year-old age group.

When asked what happened, 62 per cent said they were touched/fondled in a sensual way; 42 per cent experienced someone touching their sex organs; 37 per cent were asked to do something intimate; 33 per cent experienced masturbation; 28 per cent showed their sex organs to another person; 25 per cent were shown another person's sex organs; 24 per cent touched another person's sex organs; 21 per cent were talked to about sex in an erotic way; 21 per cent were shown pornographic material; 18 per cent touched or fondled another person in a sensual way; 16 per cent took part in oral sex; 10 per cent were flashed at in a public place; 5 per cent were involved in sexual intercourse (which could include anal sex); and 3 per cent were involved in kissing in a sensual way.

The abuser was a male stranger for 33 per cent of men. The next highest category was 'other male' for 21 per cent of our 37 men. On their questionnaires, some men specified who these men were, and they included a mixed group of people in a position of power or proximity: neighbour (mentioned twice), school barber, man in a car, football coach, stepfather, uncle's lodger and cousin (also mentioned twice).

WHO WAS THE ABUSER?	
Male stranger	33%
Other male	21%
Friend of parents	11%
Male schoolteacher	9%
Girlfriend	8%
Babysitter	8%
Other female	7%
Boyfriend	6%
Female stranger	5%
Friend of brother or sister	5%
Uncle	4%
Brother	3%
Father	3%
Female schoolteacher	2%
Don't know/prefer not to answer	9%

NSPCC figures for 1983-87 give the suspected perpetrator of sexual abuse of both boys and girls. Only 18 per cent of these cases were boys. Natural fathers were the most often implicated, followed by father substitutes and 'others'. This final category reflects the discoveries of our survey, and includes mothers' boyfriends, neighbours, lodgers and friends of the family. In 1990, parents and parent substitutes not living with the child were suspected of sexual abuse in 10 per cent of cases. These incidents usually occurred during access visits. There is also an association between a number of family characteristics and child abuse. In 30 per cent of cases, discord between the people caring for the child was the stress factor judged to have precipitated sexual abuse.

Although it has long been known that the majority of abusers are male, there has been interest recently in the issue of women sexually abusing children within their family. However, none of the 37 men in our survey cited abuse by their mother, aunt or sister. There does seem to be confusion, though, as to what constitutes abuse, given that three men cited a 'girlfriend' as the abuser.

Next we analysed the questionnaires of these 37 men to see whether their lifestyle, attitudes and sex lives differed from the general survey results. Of course, we are dealing with very small numbers here, but some behavioural patterns do emerge within this group. Of these men, 43 per cent are married; 10 per cent live with their partner; 3 per cent are widowed; 14 per cent are separated; and 30 per cent are single. Compared with men who were not abused as children, there are similar percentages of married and single men. However, this group shows a much higher divorce rate: 14 per cent are separated or divorced, in contrast to only 5 per cent of the whole sample.

According to our survey, men who were sexually abused in childhood exercise slightly less than the rest. Their alcohol intake tends to be high – they are more likely to drink two to six times a week or every day, and 30 per cent drink more than the recommended 'safe' limit, compared to only 20 per cent of non-abused men. They are also much more likely than the average man to indulge in illegal drugs: eight of them smoke marijuana (21 per cent against 7 per cent of the whole sample); three men take cocaine (8 per cent against 1 per cent) and two use aphrodisiacs (5 per cent against 1 per cent). Of the group, five have taken part in psychotherapy or psychoanalysis, two have had sex therapy and two men have had marriage counselling.

This group also have some distinctly different priorities from the sample as a whole, as this table shows.

WHAT MATTERS MOST TO ME?

RANK	FACTOR	NUMBER OF VOTES	GENERAL RANK
1.	Peace and quiet	18	=15
= 2.	Job satisfaction	15	1
= 2.	Partner	15	2
= 4.	Home	14	3
= 4.	Independence	14	4
= 4.	Freedom	14	5
7.	Health	13	= 6
= 8.	Sex	11	14
= 8.	Leisure/hobbies	11	= 6
=10.	Career	9	= 6
=10.	Female friends	9	18

For those who have been sexually abused, peace and quiet is of paramount importance, while men in the sample as a whole put it in fifteenth place. After the quiet life, the ratings follow the general pattern of other men in our survey, although sex is also more important to this group. Having been made aware of their sexuality unusually early, men who've been sexually abused tend to place sex higher in their priorities than other men. Good female companions, too, seem to be unusually important to these men.

Of this group, 29 say they are only interested in sex with women, and all but one of them describes himself as heterosexual; one man is equally attracted to women and men, and calls himself bisexual; two describe themselves as homosexual and only want sex with men; and one man says he's not interested in sex at all, but describes himself as heterosexual; another says he is only interested in sex with women, yet describes himself as asexual.

The majority of these men are only attracted to women, and describe themselves as heterosexual. However, some confusion over sexuality does exist. One man who was abused by male strangers on a few different occasions makes this comment: 'I have said that I would only have sex with women, and that in my opinion I am heterosexual. But the wording of the questions does not give scope to the possibility that under the right circumstances I would have sex with a man.' The same man leaves his options open on the question which asks which sexual activities he would definitely not like to do in the future, and does not rule out homosexual sex.

There is further confusion on the issue of sexuality within the group of four men who say they are interested in sex with women, but are also somewhat drawn towards men. Three of these men describe themselves as heterosexual, although one comments at the end of his questionnaire on his experience of oral sex with an uncle: 'I was young and it was made out to be a game, although I now feel I would like to try oral sex with a man again.'

The fourth says he doesn't know how he'd describe his sexuality, but gives the following list of attributes which he finds sexually attractive: 'Pubic hair, own body scent, male genitals, "masculine" traits, deeper voice.' The same man, when asked what form of sexual abuse he considered most serious, made this surprising remark, 'The word "serious" indicates that whatever happened was wrong. I don't consider abuse as wrong – it's normal activity.'

We examined the number of sexual partners this group have ever had, and how many they've had during the last year, to see if any significant pattern appeared.

HOW MANY SEXUAL PARTNERS HAVE YOU HAD?

	EVER		LAST YEAR	
	ABUSED MEN	NON-ABUSED MEN	ABUSED MEN	NON-ABUSED MEN
1	11%	18%	57%	68%
2-4	24%	27%	14%	16%
5-9	14%	24%	3%	3%
10-14	8%	10%	–	1%
15-19	11%	5%	–	*
20-29	3%	3%	3%	1%
30+	16%	7%	8%	1%
Can't remember	11%	7%	–	7%
None	3%	*	5%	3%
(Not stated)			(8%)	

(Note: An asterisk means less than 1 per cent.)

As with the rest of our sample, the great majority of these men have restricted themselves to one sexual partner during the last year. However, a higher percentage of men who suffered abuse as a child have had more than 30 partners overall.

This group have few problems communicating with their partner on the question of sex. As with the general sample, over two-thirds say they are able to let their sexual partner know what they want during intercourse, and that they know what their partner wants. And they have no doubt about their sexual performance: 26 out of the 36 men who've had sex say their sexual performance is either average, a little better, or much better than most. They are also believers in sexual equality: 76 per cent say both partners' sexual satisfaction is equally important.

They enjoy the same amount of sexual activity as other men in our sample, and 28 of them (76 per cent) have sex at least once a week. However, they have a tendency to masturbate more often than other men; 54 per cent of this group masturbate at least once a week, compared with 38 per cent of the whole sample.

Men's willingness to answer questions on this highly personal subject is further evidence that sexual abuse is now open for discussion. As one man commented: 'The questions on child abuse could give us an idea of how bad the problem really is.' Many of these men have normal sex lives, although there is certainly a greater degree of confusion about sexuality among this group. But it is especially revealing that men who've been sexually abused count both sex and a quiet life as particularly important.

8.

Can Men Give Women What They Want?

These are confusing times for men. Women have sexual liberation, effective contraception and higher career expectations, and many no longer rely on a man to provide a home or income. The question of exactly what women *do* want can be a worrying prospect for a man. Agony aunt Claire Rayner sums up the social revolutions that have brought us this far. 'There have been big changes over the last 30-40 years. It's the first time we've had a superfluity of men. The ratio of boy to girl babies has always been the same – 106/100 – but until the advent of modern medicine, male babies were more fragile and more died in infancy. The two World Wars compounded the problem.' It was this scarcity of men that led to the situation in the 50s where women devoured books on 'How to catch your man' and dreamed of nothing more than an ideal home and matching husband.

She continues: 'The big revolution in the Sixties wasn't the Pill but that women could pick and choose. Before that, it was any man you could get, at any price. Now women can pick from the menu. Men are confused. Many have been brought up by fathers who taught them that the biggest skill you had to learn was how to bed them without getting caught. Modern men have got to fight to get their oats. And, with the rise and acceptance of auto-eroticism and test-tube babies, women don't even need a bloke any longer. It's a terrible blow to their pride.'

Men may not always need to fight for sex, but they're certainly starting to appreciate the advantages of understanding women's needs. So we asked men what they think women look for in men. Their answers produce an intriguing picture – particularly when they are also asked to rate themselves on these attributes.

WHAT WOMEN WANT US TO BE

1.	Caring	81%
= 2.	Romantic	74%
= 2.	Fun-loving	74%
4.	Understanding	72%
5.	Sensitive	71%
6.	Treat women as equals	67%
7.	Intelligent	63%
8.	Handsome	61%
= 9.	Self-confident	57%
= 9.	Responsible	57%
11.	Strong	40%
12.	Athletic	33%
13.	In control	32%
14.	Ambitious	27%
15.	Strong-willed	18%
16.	Highly sexed	13%
17.	Upwardly mobile	12%
18.	Artistic	10%
19.	Money-orientated	9%
=20.	Macho	8%
=20.	Fearless	8%
22.	Shy	5%

According to men, women want someone who is prepared to show their emotions, yet will show them a good time. Their Top Five attributes conjure up a picture of a man who would ask his partner how her day was, cook her dinner, present her with a red rose then take her to a funfair. All the '80s' values like ambition, being macho and money-orientated, upwardly mobile and in control, come way down the list. Indeed, in the group discussions, some men felt ambition to be an old-fashioned value, and thought that the family now takes precedence.

... AND WHAT I'M LIKE

1.	Caring	80%
2.	Intelligent	68%
3.	Sensitive	66%
4.	Treat women as equals	65%
=5.	Understanding	64%
=5.	Responsible	64%
7.	Fun-loving	61%
8.	Self-confident	45%
=9.	Romantic	42%
=9.	Ambitious	42%
11.	Strong-willed	30%
=12.	Handsome	29%
=12.	In control	29%
14.	Strong	28%
15.	Athletic	27%
=16.	Highly sexed	24%
=16.	Shy	24%
18.	Artistic	16%
19.	Upwardly mobile	15%
20.	Money-orientated	15%
21.	Fearless	9%
22.	Macho	3%

However, other men in the discussion groups felt that deep down women want a man to be in control, and rated 'strong willed', 'in control' and 'responsible' as very important. 'It's possibly an old cliché, but I do think that women look to men to be in control and be the decision-maker,' said a married 31 year old. 'I do feel I go out from the cave, hunt, bring food back. There are genetic differences.' But despite such references to Neanderthal man, they all felt that women didn't want macho men, but would rather have men who were caring and understanding.

As far as men's self-assessment of their characteristics is concerned, there's a huge drop between the 61 per cent who believe they're fun-loving, to the 45 per cent of the sample who say they're self-confident. Even fewer believe they are romantic. Three out of four men believe that women want romance from a man, yet few can deliver this quality: only 42 per cent say they are romantic at heart, with single men rating themselves much higher than those who are married. In the discussion groups, some men seemed proud of the fact that they weren't romantic, viewing it as boring and effeminate, or of strictly short-term value. 'I'm not romantic. I wouldn't normally buy my wife flowers unless I was late or had done something wrong. I might think, shit, I'll have to pop to Safeways for a bag of flowers or a box of chocolates or something,' said a married 32 year old.

Two in five men think women want a man to be strong, while a third believe athleticism holds a certain appeal. Only 10 per cent say women appreciate artistic men, and even fewer think they want men who are macho, fearless or shy.

Men in our sample also seem to think being highly sexed is pretty unimportant to women: 13 per cent rate it as an attractive quality. In the groups, men confirmed that in their experience, most women don't want men who constantly have sex on their mind: suggesting that they felt they were a little too highly sexed for their partner's liking.

Where self-confidence is concerned, although most groups of men reckon it's a quality women value, there are significant differences in the extent to which they believe they possess it. The highest earners have the most confidence in themselves, while those currently without a steady relationship are relatively lacking in confidence. Self-confidence is particularly high among men who have had the most sexual partners and began their sexual careers comparatively young.

Men who have had the most partners are more convinced than men with fewer conquests that women want them to be romantic, understanding, caring and fun-loving. However, they also tend to think women value upward mobility and ambition: 33 per cent of these men rate ambition, compared with 24 per cent of men with only one partner, so their tactics seem to have been successful!

Older men rate practically all of these attributes as less important than the younger men. Men under 24 are significantly more likely to rate the following qualities more highly: being strong, ambitious, highly sexed, fun-loving, handsome, artistic and shy. Men with basic education and those earning over £25k

MEN ON SEX are more convinced of the importance to women of a man being in control. The idea that a woman wants to be treated as an equal is more likely to be dismissed by men in their early 30s.

Men at the top and bottom of the employment heap have some interesting clashes in their points of view. Men in management think self-confidence is the way to a girl's heart, along with being strong-willed, romantic, intelligent and upwardly mobile. In other words, they rate their own characteristics as particularly attractive to the opposite sex! On the other hand, some unemployed men think women are after a man who's highly sexed and handsome, but not particularly responsible. These men are confident they are highly sexed, artistically skilled and irresponsible – so on those scores they feel they can satisfy women's needs. But not one of the unemployed men thinks he's money-orientated.

There's an inverse correlation between sex and sensitivity: men who are currently having the *least* sex rate themselves as most sensitive, and are most likely to say sensitivity is what a woman wants. On the other hand, men who have the most sex have more faith in the power of the 80s values already mentioned: being strong, ambitious, macho, and upwardly mobile. They are also more likely than other men to say women want someone who's highly sexed. However, as the following table shows, only half of the men having the most sex think they're highly sexed!

ARE YOU HIGHLY SEXED?

SEXUAL ACTIVITY	
4 plus times a week	50%
2-3 days a week	23%
1 day a week	23%
Once or twice a month	21%
Less than once a month	20%
Never	16%

Single men are generally likely to believe women want strong, ambitious, upwardly mobile men who are fixated on money, while rating themselves slightly more ambitious and upwardly mobile than average. In their view, women are more interested in a man who's fun-loving than one who's responsible, and their self-rating matches up to this standard. In their own opinion, single men tend to be handsome, romantic, shy and understanding, and are less reluctant than the rest to describe themselves as artistic.

Men in a regular relationship consider that women want a caring, intelligent, sensitive sort of chap. As far as they're concerned, women value understanding and are keen on equality. Slightly more self-confident, strong-willed and in control than most, they are more likely to think they treat women as equals than men with occasional relationships, no relationships or the two-timers.

Men who have occasional relationships tend to think women rate the strong competitive instinct in men, rather than caring, sensitive qualities. In their view, women are after a man who's fun-loving and romantic, and this is basically how they see themselves. They think it's less important to women for men to be understanding and treat women as equals.

The more sexual experience a man has, the more likely he is to say that women want ambitious, upwardly mobile men. Men who've had more than four partners also tend to say women like a man who's fun-loving, athletic and romantic: the type who'd jump on to a waterbed with a rose between his teeth. Men who've had more sexual partners are more convinced that women want to be understood and think their partners value a caring attitude more than equality. Those who've had between five and nine partners are more likely to say women want a man who's highly sexed *and* responsible (a man with an erection and a condom perhaps). The group of men who've had more than ten partners think they're particularly strong and ambitious, but don't rate themselves as shy. Compared with men who've stuck to one woman, they rate themselves as much more handsome, self-confident and strong-willed. They also see themselves as more fearless and in control. Seventy-five per cent of these men think they're clever, compared with only 64 per cent of men who've had just the one partner.

Men who've had more than five sexual partners are also much more likely to consider themselves highly sexed than those who have only had one partner. Just 17 per cent of 'One-Woman Men' say they're highly sexed, compared with 30 per cent of those who've had between five and nine partners, and 38 per cent of men who've had sex with more than ten women.

There are similar patterns relating to how often a man has sex. Men having sex at least four times a week are much more likely than those having sex less frequently to say women want strong,

MEN ON SEX

macho, money-orientated men. In contrast, they also feel women put a high value on understanding and equality. They're the group most likely to believe women want a man to be highly sexed: 28 per cent of them say this. Given their high level of sexual activity, this says something for their powers of persuasion! Half of them describe themselves as ambitious, and they also think they're stronger and more upwardly mobile and fun loving than men having less sex, but not that responsible. The most confident and sure of their looks, they see themselves as strong-willed and in control.

So what *do* women want? Imagine three men – one with a vibrator, the next brandishing a whip and the third holding a massive ear trumpet. Chronicler of eroticism and poet Fiona Pitt-Kethley has no doubts which man she'd find most attractive. 'The ability to listen is one of the most vital factors for good sex. A lot of classic good looks turn me on; I wouldn't fancy an ugly or old man – I'm quite caddish in that respect. A sense of humour can help a man with less good looks. If he talks well and listens well, he gets a lot of extra points.'

For swimming star Sharron Davies, fit men hold more of an appeal: 'I find men who bother with their physique more of a turn-on. You walk better, hold yourself upright, smile more. A lot of men could be more sexy if they got fit, because it helps an awful lot with self-esteem.' Looks are also an important consideration: 'I actually go for tall, dark and smouldering men. My pin-up type is Tom Selleck because he's very much a man. I know there was that thing about him being gay, but he's still very sexy. There's a German decathlete, a doctor called Siggy Wentz – he's my perfect package: intelligent, sporty, good sense of humour, nice eyes.'

MEASURING UP

We asked men how well equipped they are for sex, both physically and mentally. Forty-four per cent of men don't know if they are well endowed; 32 per cent say they're not; and 24 per cent say they are. The older a man is, the more likely he is to say he's got a small penis: 44 per cent of men over 40 say they're not well endowed, compared with only 19 per cent of men under 24. However, about half of the youngest men say they don't know how they measure up, and as a man gets older, he becomes progressively less unsure and more sure he's on the small side. Time will tell, it seems.

Men in the discussion groups tended to agree that most of them wouldn't say they were well endowed, because they couldn't be sure. A married 27 year old gave another reason: 'Most people here have probably seen a sex film – most of the guys there have 12-inch dicks, if you want to put it crudely.'

Half the single men don't know if they're well endowed, whereas those who are separated are most likely to say they've got what it takes. A man's confidence seems to rise with the number of relationships he has on the go: 36 per cent of the two-timers brag that they're well endowed, compared with only 16 per cent of men who aren't currently in a relationship. Single men are generally the most likely to say they don't know whether or not they're well endowed.

At the opposite end of the spectrum, experience breeds confidence. Men who've had more than ten partners are much more likely than men who've had fewer partners to say they're well endowed, while half the men who've stuck to one woman don't know whether they are or not. Having lots of sex also tends to convince men they're blessed in the trouser department, whereas men who have sex between once a week and once a month are the most likely to say they're less well favoured. And 56 per cent of men who never have sex don't know what to think. Men who think they're big boys are more likely to have lost their virginity early and enjoyed it a great deal the first time. However, those who found losing their virginity a fairly miserable experience are more likely to say they're not well endowed.

Does Size Matter?

Not according to 60 per cent of the men. Twenty-one per cent say it does, and 20 per cent don't know. The idea that 21 per cent think size does matter was cause for some anxiety in the discussion groups, where most men thought it wasn't an issue. As a cohabiting 30 year old said: 'Most women I've known give the impression it's not the size of it, it's what you do with it.' This opinion was backed up by a cohabiting 24-year-old manager: 'It's drummed into us – whether you read problem pages or whatever – from an early age, that it *isn't* important.'

Those who have sex most often and the men who've had more than ten partners are the most likely to say size matters, while those who have a moderate amount of sex tend to think it doesn't.

MEN ON SEX

Men in their late 30s believe that size isn't an issue, while 26 per cent of men earning over £25k say it is important to women. Married and separated men are more likely than cohabiting or single men to say women aren't interested in the size of a man's penis. Men with occasional relationships are more likely to think women do take it into consideration. Having established that they tend to think they're well endowed, men having the most sex and those who've had the most partners are the most confident that size matters. Whereas men who've had between two and nine partners and those having an average amount of sex are likely to say it isn't an issue.

PILLOW TALK

We asked a final question about what men believe women want – in bed.

TOP TEN BETWEEN THE SHEETS	
1. Affection	72%
2. Tenderness	65%
3. Sensuality	61%
4. Passion	57%
5. Stamina	29%
6. Energy	21%
7. A dominant man	15%
8. A submissive man	2%
9. No idea	2%
10. Don't care	2%

A yawning chasm opens up after the first four attributes, with men giving little credence to the idea that women want stamina and energy. It seems men would rather believe women need hugs and emotion than raw, steamy sex that goes on for hours. In small group discussions, the consensus was that women and men have different priorities in sex. Both want to make love, but it's men who are more interested in having sex. The distinction between the two is linked to men's belief that women are after emotional closeness as much as physical pleasure, and that women regard the sexual act as something that should be protracted rather than completed as briskly as possible.

Some men also drew a distinction between different types of relationships. They felt that whereas affection and tenderness are meaningful in the context of a long-term relationship, an affair might demand other qualities! 'It depends totally whether it was in a relationship or out of one. If it was outside – then passion and stamina!' said a single 27 year old. And different situations also make different demands: 'I don't think that every time it has to fulfil the same set of criteria,' said a single 30 year old. 'Sometimes it could be tenderness and foreplay, perhaps the candle-lit dinner idea. Whereas other times it could be just the quickie – spontaneous, spur of the moment, a quick bang, for want of a better word.'

According to our sample there are different opinions on affection and tenderness in the various age groups. The youngest men put affection at the top of their list, with its overtones of friendliness and warmth. However, men in their 40s say tenderness – implying a sense of vulnerability – is more important to a woman. Young men also put a lot more faith in passion and sensuality than older men, and are the most likely to say dominant men appeal to women. It's not surprising to find that young men at their sexual peak put a higher value on stamina and energy than the older generation, which considers them much less important.

The most educated men are among the least likely to say women want affection or stamina in bed. Perhaps any woman who ends up in bed with a man earning over £25k shouldn't expect much passion or energy, and it's the lowest earners who are most likely to offer them stamina. Whereas 80 per cent of men in lower forms of employment say affection is by far the most important attribute.

Only 52 per cent of married men think passion is what women want in bed, compared with 63 per cent of single men! Married men believe in affection instead, and place little value in stamina or energy. Eighty-four per cent of separated men say tenderness is vital, while single men are among the most likely to say passion is important. They also have relatively high ratings for stamina and energy.

If a man is in a regular relationship, he's most likely to say affection in bed is what matters most to women. The idea that

MEN ON SEX women like submissive men is only taken up by 2 per cent of our sample.

Having had a greater number of partners leads a man to value affection slightly less highly, and raw passion and sensuality more highly. Men who've had more than ten partners are also among the most likely to say women like men who are dominant in bed and can prove their stamina! The men having the most sex are most inclined to believe women want affection, followed by passion and sensuality, with tenderness less important. They are also great enthusiasts of the idea that dominance, stamina and energy appeal to women.

The start of a man's sexual career seems to affect his attitude towards what women want in bed. The more he enjoyed losing his virginity, the more likely he is to say sensuality appeals to the opposite sex.

In conclusion, men do seem pretty sure they know what women want. But this doesn't necessarily mean they're prepared to adapt their behaviour accordingly. Although only a quarter think they're well hung, the majority believe that women don't mind. It seems that, if all else fails, men can always rely on the confidence trick.

9.

Let's Talk About Sex

Some men in the discussion groups seemed to see men and women on opposite sides of a great divide, both with different needs and different forms of expression. According to poet Fiona Pitt-Kethley, it doesn't have to be this way. 'The assumption that there are vast mental and emotional differences between men and women drives a wedge between sexes. I think there are many points of resemblance. The essential problem with British sexuality is that we live in a very prudish society, so we don't talk about sex. That's the root of our problems.'

However, men in our discussion groups showed little reluctance to talk candidly about sex. The results of our questionnaire certainly provoked some strong reactions, and here are their comments on the subject of sexual performance, communication and fidelity.

HIGH PERFORMERS

On the subject of sexual performance, men appear a confident lot! Most rate their own sexual performance as average or better: 11 per cent believe it's a lot better than most, 17 per cent say a little better, and 39 per cent rate themselves about average. Only 3 per cent rate themselves below average – and all these 'a little worse than most'; only two men rated themselves 'a lot worse than most'. However, quite a high number of men (29 per cent) ticked the 'don't know' box on this question, presumably feeling unable to judge their performance.

The men interviewed in small groups confirmed this basic state of affairs: some argued that it was impossible really to 'know' how good you are in bed (although it was undoubtedly a subject of interest); but most appeared to feel that they stacked up pretty well in performance terms. Some pointed out that the main means of judging your performance consists of comments made by partners; and these are more than likely to be complimentary, if only because a partner knows that's what men like to hear. One divorced 37 year old in the South East wrote at the end of his questionnaire: 'I have always received flattering comments. . . . However, knowing that women generally tend to flatter, I take this with a pinch of salt. Despite comments such as "fantastic" and "out of this world," I am also aware that my next partner may not be so easily impressed.' A 19 year old from Surrey was also wary of taking positive comments at face value: 'A lot of the time women will comment on how good you are, you'll get a letter from them the next day or something. But it's in their best interests for them to say it was great.'

Some men in the group discussions felt that, in the context of a long-term relationship, if you and your partner had a mutually enjoyable sex life, you would be inclined to feel confident about your performance – despite the impossibility of comparing it with any 'norm'. As one 32 year old put it: 'On the performance side, it's how sex is with your partner, isn't it, and you know whether it's good, bad or indifferent. And if you enjoy it and she enjoys it, you tend to think it's better than most.'

Few men in the group discussions were willing to admit to vulnerability in sexual situations, except occasionally when looking back on early experiences. There was no mention of impotence, and a strong implication that men were nearly always 'ready for action'. It may well be that group discussions are not the right forum for voicing fears and inadequacies on the subject of sex, or it may be that the men who chose to participate in such groups were more than averagely confident. Men with such doubts might also perhaps be less willing to complete questionnaires on the subject.

According to the survey, the men most confident of their performance were the most experienced (in terms of numbers of partners), those who had sex most frequently, and those who had lost their virginity early. Others more inclined to say their performance is a lot better than most are men with basic education, those in lower forms of employment, separated men and the two-timers. Those not currently in a relationship were less confident.

Men who'd only ever had one partner were particularly likely to say they didn't know how their performance compared.

THE VOICE OF EXPERIENCE

All the men in the group discussions felt that they were better lovers than they had been in the past – it seemed as if all experience was good experience, in the sense of increasing learning and sensitivity. Over time they had become more relaxed, especially in the context of a long-term relationship. The anxiety factor faded as one got to know somebody – but this was a retrospective observation, in that it seemed that when younger, they had not felt dogged by a lack of confidence at the time (perhaps because at this stage their general keenness for sex overshadowed all!).

Men said that it was possible to learn either through having a number of different relationships, or within one long-term relationship. Being a good lover could mean you understood 'women' – or that you had grown to understand your particular woman. One 37 year old who'd been married for 17 years said: 'I think I have a better sex life now than I did when I was 18 – I think I get more out of it, it's more pleasurable. . . . It's probably because I've got a greater understanding of my wife and myself. It's a learning process.'

But men also put a lot of store by the idea of sexual chemistry between two people: thus you could be a good lover (i.e. have a great sex life) with one person, but be a lousy lover with another. 'I've been to bed with a number of girls, and some of them you come away thinking that was crap, and others you come away from thinking that was really nice, and we had a whale of a time, sort of thing. It's the combination and chemistry of two people, not one person being able to shag solidly for three hours,' said a cohabiting 25 year old. Factors such as mood and alcohol intake were also acknowledged to influence performance.

HOW WAS IT FOR YOU?

The survey suggests that men are better at letting their partners know what they themselves would like than they are at eliciting from partners what *they* would like. Eighty-four per cent of those surveyed are confident they can let their partner know what they want to happen, 9 per cent aren't sure and 7 per cent say that they can't. The most confident of all are those in their 30s, and those who have sex four or more times a week. Among the least confident on this issue are those without regular partners.

When asked how confident they are of knowing what their sexual partners want, the majority (59 per cent) describe themselves as 'fairly' confident. Twenty-eight per cent are very confident, and most of the rest not very confident. Confidence about partners' wants correlates with more experience, higher frequency of sex, early loss of virginity, and being a father. Younger men tend to be slightly less confident overall, and this was confirmed in the groups. Men in their 30s looked back on their experiences when younger as being full of mystery while lacking communication. They noted that, crucially, women's orgasms are less 'clear cut' than men's, in that there is no obvious evidence equivalent to ejaculation. As one married 37 year old put it: 'Women's satisfaction is a mysterious affair when you're younger. We were all the same then, no two ways about that. You knew what the end result was from your point of view, but you never really knew what it was from theirs. Until you settled down with one partner and had more experiences.' A 28-year-old single man expressed similar sentiments: 'Women are still a mystery to men sexually. Apparently, so we're told, medically, sexual pleasure for women is much greater. But I know for a fact that most men are mystified by the way a woman works, as far as erogenous zones, as far as orgasms and so on are concerned.'

Men's satisfaction was more straightforward. As one cohabiting 39 year old put it, 'From a man's point of view, satisfaction is just a matter of time.' Some felt that, unlike men, women could be sexually satisfied without achieving orgasm. But a 19-year-old student saw the situation as a case of women being more demanding than men: "I think it's far easier to fulfil a man than it is to fulfil a woman. The requirement's less for a man. I think women can be quite selfish in sexual relationships, they can be more greedy.'

SEX TALK

The men in the groups identified communication during sex as a sensitive issue. Some spoke of the question, 'What would you like me to do?' invariably being answered with, 'Whatever you like.' This could be interpreted as evasive – a partner not *daring* to say what she would like – but such reticence was felt to be more common on the part of men, some of whom gave the distinct impression they would be up for more 'deviant' practices. However, they felt wives or girlfriends would be less amenable. A cohabiting 22 year old said: 'There might be things – kinky things – you wouldn't tell her because she's your partner, I suppose. If she said no, you'd feel a right prick! You have to live with that person after.'

There was also the possibility that a woman might genuinely not know what she wanted. Men pointed out that 'steps forward' in sexual understanding often happened inadvertently – a couple might 'stumble across' an activity or position that gave particular pleasure. 'It's very hard for people to talk beyond the basics,' said one cohabiting 24 year old: 'I'd imagine there aren't very many open relationships after only a couple of years. I imagine it takes time. And very often things can be found out by accident.' Certainly one of the benefits of a long-term relationship was felt to be a good mutual understanding of what turned the other person on.

However, some, like this single man aged 30, argued that communication could become more difficult as time went on, if preferences weren't made clear at the beginning: 'I can see it's possible that if in the opening year or two you've never really found out what the other person likes, it must become more and more impossible to say . . . and you get to the point where it's – he's always done that and I've never liked it.'

Some might argue that men just don't have the vocabulary to express their feelings. 'The way society brings boys up is tragic, and leads to their problems in expressing themselves,' according to a single 25 year old. 'Men find it very difficult to communicate with their partners in a majority of cases. They find it very difficult to accept their feminine side. When relationships end, women tend to recover quicker, because they go and talk about it with their friends. Men bottle things up and become bitter and angry.'

SATISFIED NOW?

According to 74 per cent of men, their own and their partner's sexual satisfaction are equally important. Of the others, however, nearly eight times as many (23 per cent) believe that their partner's satisfaction is more important than the percentage (only 3 per cent) who believe their own is. Those who had more than one sexual partner on the go were more inclined to put emphasis on their partners' satisfaction.

In the group discussions some of the men found it difficult to distinguish between partners' satisfaction and their own: to many, turning someone else on was in itself the biggest turn-on of all. A married 35 year old commented: 'You could answer that your partner's satisfaction is more important to you, but in a way, giving your partner satisfaction gives *you* satisfaction.' Younger men agreed. A single 27 year old said: 'The most exciting thing in sex, and I think most men would agree with this, is turning somebody else on. That's the most stimulating thing.' Or, as a student of 19 put it: 'I can turn myself on. It's far more fun turning someone else on.'

Again, there was the implication that a man's satisfaction (or at least orgasm) is a 'given', whereas a woman's is more elusive. Therefore if a woman is satisfied, the act is more likely to have been satisfactory overall. It's almost as if a woman's satisfaction is more of a challenge, and hence, when it occurs, more of an achievement. This was the perspective of a cohabiting 39 year old: 'I know that I can gain satisfaction from sex, and with that knowledge I would like to enter it (to coin a phrase!) feeling that I could give my partner as much satisfaction as myself. Just by *initiating* the act I know I'm going to get my satisfaction.'

Giving a woman satisfaction might also reap future rewards. 'It's a turn-on that she's turned on, and it has a knock-on effect,' began one married 37 year old, 'and there's the added bonus – if your partner enjoyed it, then next time you fancy a bit, you're quids in!'

LOVE AND THE QUICKIE

In all the groups men drew a distinction between sex and making love. 'There's sex and making love definitely,' said a married 27 year old, 'and I think most women would prefer it the romantic way . . . rather than just in the kitchen, over the sink or whatever, like *Fatal Attraction*.' On a simple level it was often said that women like making love – men do too, but men also sometimes like pure sex. Making love was also equated with being more romantic and taking more time; 'sex' was a faster, more urgent process – sometimes associated with places other than bed! 'Sex in the shower isn't love, is it?' said a 31 year old. One married 30 year old saw it as 'a terminology problem: women want to make love, men want to have sex, or have a quickie, or whatever. Making love takes longer than having sex.'

It seemed as if men sometimes used the sex versus making love distinction to avoid having to think too deeply how to satisfy their partner physically as well as mentally. Men were happier to perceive their sexual inadequacies as emotional rather than physical. It was easier for them to believe that women want affection and tenderness than for them to think too hard about women's nitty-gritty physical needs. Many men, especially the more 'macho' types, didn't mind at all admitting shortcomings on the emotional front – it was almost a celebration of their maleness. According to a married 27 year old: 'I don't know if most men are romantic enough to turn the woman on. Talking to my wife over these situations, I get the argument thrown back at me. If I was a bit more tender, a bit more loving, a bit more gentle, took more time, it might be different. Whereas I'm sort of rush rush rush, let's get it over and done with and let's go to sleep.' A cohabiting 30 year old also saw the situation as men having their 'needs', which had little to do with making love: 'The way we are, males, with our hormone levels, makes us want more, and to be more spontaneous – we want a quick orgasm. At certain points when you haven't had it for a while, it's like Vesuvius going off – you've just got to have an orgasm.'

In some relationships it seemed that women accepted men's physical needs as a separate issue from their own, and would 'give' men sex almost as a present or reward. For a number of these couples, this did appear to be a workable pattern. As one 27-year-old married man said: 'She's not as keen and not as bothered, but she knows I am keen and I am bothered, and perhaps if I've taken her out, or done the washing up she'll make sure that I have more of a good time than perhaps she does. And we just treat it that way, and it works quite well in a funny sort of way.' But a single 27 year old said he'd felt short-changed by being 'given' sex by his girlfriend: 'The very obvious, very apparent thing of making a man ejaculate isn't necessarily giving him sexual satisfaction. I mean it's easy to equate the two, "because the guy has come, he's had a good time", but it's not necessarily the case. In fact somebody can do that to you and make you feel really let down – oh God, he wants a fuck again, quickly get it over with, and he'll go back to sleep. You can end up feeling – hang on, I wanted to make love, but we've just had sex.'

There were some more 'liberated' men who refused to view women as never wanting 'sex'. A single 29 year old thought: 'Women probably want sex far more often than men think they do. I should have thought there are plenty of women who just want sex for the sake of it, who see a bloke and think, whoah, wouldn't mind him!' Some relationships clearly had room for both sex and making love – sometimes one was more appropriate, sometimes the other. One 31-year-old man described the situation in his, seemingly happy, marriage: 'There's a time and a place. My wife and I sometimes have sex and we know it's just sex. It's a physical thing. There is *some* love there, but there are other times when there's more emotion.' In relationships where making love was frequent and satisfying, the woman was often more open to interspersing lovemaking with occasions of pure sex. Perhaps it's fears of prostitution and being 'used' that cause some women to find pure sex distasteful – and in a good relationship where such fears would be out of place, the woman is happier to abandon herself to the purely physical from time to time.

There were also a number of men who had come to believe that perhaps a more traditionally 'female' approach to making love was in fact altogether more satisfying for both parties. They tended to view themselves as having 'learned' that taking more time, having more protracted periods of foreplay and so on, was in the long term more rewarding. On one level it was expressed by this 31 year old as, 'The more you put into it, the more you get out of it as well.' A single 28 year old was more specific: 'You learn that it's not just diving in, you learn just simple things, like stroking and kissing, not necessarily focusing on genitals.'

WHERE DID YOU LEARN THAT?

When men in the survey are asked how they acquired their sexual technique, 74 per cent cite their sexual partners. Among the 35-39 year olds, this figure is as high as 81 per cent. After sexual partners, the next highest score is 'conversations with male friends', but this is only 27 per cent. In the groups men reported that conversations among men were not famous for their honesty, but that they could increase general awareness of sexual possibilities. As a married 39 year old said: 'Conversations with men aren't particularly frank, they tend to be bragging and strutting, but you do get to know of other practices – "haven't you done

. . .," "didn't you do . . .," and so on.'

Twenty-three per cent of men think that TV, films, video, or radio have influenced their sexual technique, 18 per cent say sex manuals, text-books or technique books, and 13 per cent mention conversations with female friends. Seven per cent cite sex education at school. Only 2 per cent think conversations with parents were of any significance.

The survey shows that younger men are more likely than older to say they have learned from conversations with both male and female friends, and from TV, films, radio or videos. Divorced and separated men, those with a regular sexual partner plus other(s), and those with a high level of sexual activity are particularly likely to say they had learned their technique from sexual partners. Men who have lost their virginity late have a greater tendency to cite sex manuals and other books.

FIDELITY V. NOVELTY

In the groups, happily married men with children clearly saw fidelity as part of their lives; although not immune to other women's charms, they were not prepared to jeopardise what they had for the sake of a few hours of passion. In the words of a married 37 year old: 'If you've got a stable relationship, it's a big risk for one or two nights of fun. I can always go home feeling keen and fulfil my fantasies at home.' A married 30 year old said that, when it came to the crunch, he'd managed to resist temptation: 'I've had opportunities, and I've been very close to taking them, but I've usually got out of the car or whatever. I'd feel guilty – you'd have to live with yourself after.'

But most married men in the groups did feel there was no harm in looking at other women – being mentally unfaithful – and thought their wives probably felt the same way. For some of these men, chatting a woman up is enough: it proves they can still play the game, without threatening their marriage, and was seen as perfectly natural. They certainly did not think it was a sign of dissatisfaction with their partner. 'Most blokes – if they're out with the lads on a stag night or something – there aren't many who wouldn't chat some woman up,' according to a married 30 year old. 'When you're married, it's more of an ego trip. They naturally assume you're not trying to chat them up to get off with them. You can spend a whole evening chatting them up and get off on that. And you wander off at the end thinking – I can still do it.'

This view was confirmed by a married 33 year old: 'I sometimes think, I wonder what it's like with that person, whether they're passionate. I must admit there was somebody I thought about after I met her and something clicked – a bit of brief eye contact. And then you think – if I was young and free again . . .'

The younger men who had just started living with their partner were those who debated fidelity and its problems most passionately. For them, there is a clear trade-off: a comfortable home life and love, for the thrill of the chase, and all the novelty and excitement that entails. 'When I was young, as long as I had enough money in my pocket, I didn't give a shit,' said a cohabiting 26 year old. 'But now I've got a house, I want to build it up, start a family, things like that. That may be more important than chasing loads of women around.' There was a common feeling that priorities changed with time, as a single 29 year old put it: 'You do get a bit cheesed off with going to bed with the same person all the time, but less so than when I was 19.' Some of the slightly older men looked wistfully back on their wild youth, but also felt that they had different values now, and that there were definite benefits to long-term relationships.

Many still longed for that thrill, and would chat women up as a means of recreating the kick of being in pursuit of a woman. In the words of a cohabiting 25 year old: 'Curiosity plays a big part and the challenge of the chase, to know that you can still do it.' A cohabiting 30 year old agreed that the desire remains: 'I suspect that even if you're cohabiting, most men would still fancy someone in the office, or chat someone up in the pub.'

It did seem, though, that these men rarely actually went to bed with the women they pursued, although that could at times be a knife-edge situation. A few admitted that they might be persuaded, in certain circumstances. A 24 year old living with his partner had even convinced himself that an affair could benefit his relationship. 'Having sex on the side doesn't necessarily mean you love your partner less. It sometimes works to make you love them more.' However, for some of those contemplating this move, a double standard prevailed. 'I suppose, even now, if the chance presented itself, I'd take it,' said a cohabiting 33 year old. 'But if she did, I'd go up the wall.'

For the youngest men, long-term fidelity held little charm. They wanted to experiment with lots of partners and viewed the idea of being tied down with horror. 'I'm only 19 – I definitely know I wouldn't want to miss out on what I'm going through at the moment – having a bloody good time, no responsibility,' said one, concluding: 'I don't want to commit myself to any relationship like marriage.' In the light of this fear of commitment, it's not surprising that many young men found the pursuit of women the most exciting part. 'The chase is better than the kill. I can desire a girl, but once I've got her, I'm not so interested,' said a single 19 year old.

Another 19 year old regretted the period spent in a steady relationship as time 'missed'. ' I went out with someone for two years – started when I was 17 and finished a few months ago – and it's the best thing I ever did, to get out of that relationship. I still *seek* relationships, I think everybody does, but when I'm in them I want out very quickly.'

Some of the younger men felt that having a wild period in their youth, more or less screwing everything that moved, was an important part of their sexual development, and laid more stable foundations for fidelity later. However, this was not the case according to several of the men who had married early. They felt they may possibly have missed out, but perhaps were more devoted to their partners, or felt threatened by the idea of other relationships. One man who married at the age of 21 described how a fantasy partner took the edge off his dissatisfaction at missing out on other relationships. 'I used to use "the other woman," not a real one you understand. She was called Sandra – a fantasy woman. My wife knew about it,' said a married 33 year old. ' I did get married very young – I'd known my wife since I was 17. I don't regret it, else I wouldn't have everything I've now got, but the fantasy was a way of satisfying that frustration.'

Overall, it seems that the majority of men have a certain confidence about sex: they feel they can communicate their needs fairly well, and rate their own performance pretty highly. Women's sexuality is in some fundamental way regarded as more complex than men's, and women's satisfaction remains something of a mystery to younger men, but understanding of female needs can be reached through a long-term relationship. Women may be categorised as wanting to 'make love' rather than have sex, but in truth many men also find 'making love' more satisfactory. However, in good relationships there is room for both. And fidelity? Well, for men in our group discussions, it seems that's just a part of growing up.

10.

Dream Girls

Given that well-known statistic that men think about sex once every ten minutes, it is perhaps surprising that only 72 per cent of our sample say they fantasise about having sex with someone they haven't slept with. By contrast, all the men in the groups said they had fantasies. Perhaps they were using a wider definition than men in the sample, to include the most fleeting of thoughts.

FLIGHTS OF FANTASY

The men most likely to daydream about sex are the young and the unemployed. Men with higher education are also more prone to fantasy than those with fewer qualifications: only 60 per cent of men who left school at 16 say they have sexual fantasies, compared to 77 per cent of men who prolonged their studies further.

If a man is attached, it seems to cut down on his fantasising. Married and cohabiting men are much less inclined to think about sex than those who are separated or single, and only 67 per cent of men with a regular relationship find time to fantasise, compared with 86 per cent of men with occasional relationships. In one of the groups, a married 33 year old agreed with this finding: 'I should think fantasies are important to those people without a regular partner, because in order to get a partner you must role-play the scene beforehand. You can't just go blindly in there.' Fantasising is also less common for men with very young children: only 59 per cent of these men say they fantasise about sex with someone they haven't slept with.

Men who've had the most partners are much more prone to fantasy than those who've been faithful to one woman; the figures are 81 per cent and 63 per cent respectively. However, it's men who are currently have very little or no sexual activity who fantasise the most. According to a single 27 year old, the benefits depend on your state of mind: 'I think if you're feeling alone and unloved, fantasies can depress you. But if that's not the case, it can be good for you, if you're bored.' And Claire Rayner believes that fantasies really can be better than sex! 'The best sex is in your head, anyway. Fantasy has been part of human imagery since the year dot. If you only have sex with your genitals, it's a very poor thing.'

We asked men which occasions and locations they find most conducive to fantasy.

WHERE AND WHEN?

While lying in bed	69%
While having a bath/shower	36%
While socialising in a pub/at a party	35%
While watching television/films	34%
At work, but not at meetings	32%
While driving/travelling (not to work)	28%
While driving/travelling to work	25%
Sometimes, when having sex with my regular partner	22%
During meetings at work	12%
While talking on the telephone	9%
Always, when having sex with my regular partner	2%
Other	5%

The finding that fantasising occurs most often in bed didn't surprise a married 27 year old in one of the groups. 'I should think lying in bed had a high score,' he said. 'It goes back to the boredom thing. You go to bed and you think – what can I think about? And it's up periscope!'

Men in the discussion groups agreed that being in bed or the bath are prime times for fantasy; you're relaxed, and masturbation is certainly more of a possibility here than if you're in a meeting at work!

Men who spent a lot of time long-distance driving also felt this was a key time for the fleeting fantasy. For this married 32 year old, just getting behind the wheel is enough to start a sexual train of thought: 'I always think of sex when I'm driving. When I'm stuck in a traffic jam and I see a nice bird in a car – nothing turns me on more! There's something sexy about shoulders and a head.' Our survey shows it's men in their late 30s who are most likely to have drive-time fantasies.

In the discussion groups, a married 43 year old described how he finds the television a source of inspiration for fantasies: 'You get plenty of images off the television without having to look at porno mags or anything. You just can't help having moments of fantasy.'

Only 1 per cent of married men *always* fantasise about someone else when they're having sex with their wives. However, they are the group most likely to say they sometimes do: 31 per cent occasionally think about someone else. In the small group discussions, it was interesting to find that dissatisfied married men had the more elaborate and 'possible' fantasies – usually about someone they knew.

Men under 30 are by far the most likely to fantasise in a pub or at a party, and men under 35 are much more prone to fantasising in bed than older men. But very few of the youngest in our survey tend to fantasise about another woman during sex with their partner. However, men over 40 are more likely to experience flights of fancy at this time.

For many men, their late 20s are a time to focus on forging ahead with a career. But according to our survey, their thoughts are not always on business when they're at work! Forty-two per cent of these men think about sex at work, and 16 per cent carry on dreaming during work meetings as well.

Men in their early 30s like thinking dirty on the phone, as do 17 per cent of men earning over £25k. The richest men also particularly like thinking about sex during meetings at work, when they're driving and sometimes during sex with their partner.

Letting your thoughts drift at a party, in a pub or while watching TV is particularly common among the unemployed and men whose education ended at the age of 16. Single men are also prone to fantasy while drinking or partying, and are big fans of fantasy on the phone and in bed. Unemployed men seem keen on fantasising when they're in bed or driving around, but rarely during sex with their main squeeze.

It makes sense that those most likely to be having sex in bed are the least likely to be found lying there thinking about it. As the following table shows, only 58 per cent of men who have sex more than four times a week fantasise while lying in bed, compared to 85 per cent of men who never have sex.

DO YOU FANTASISE ABOUT SEX LYING IN BED?

LEVEL OF ACTIVITY	
4 plus days a week	58%
2-3 days a week	62%
Once a week	64%
Once or twice a month	69%
Less than once a month	82%
Never	85%

Similarly, having a regular relationship leaves less time for fantasy, since these men are the least likely to fantasise while lying in bed. But 89 per cent of men with no relationship do think about sex when they're in bed. These men also like fantasising when driving (but not when they're going to work!), but rarely get excited on the phone. In contrast, men with occasional relationships tend to think about sex at work, while socialising and in bed.

Men who've had more than ten sexual partners are among the most likely to drift into fantasy land during work meetings. They also tend to think about sex more than most when they're driving and on the phone. But it's the men who've had between five and nine partners who find it hardest to keep their thoughts on the woman in bed with them: 30 per cent of these men sometimes pretend they're having sex with someone else. These are also the men to watch at work – 39 per cent say they daydream about sex on the job. Fantasising about sex while in the bath is favoured by men who've had fewer partners; this is a prime location for 42 per cent of those who've had between two and four partners.

The more sex a man has, the more likely he is to be thinking of someone else at the time! A third of men with the highest sexual activity sometimes find their thoughts are elsewhere, but this only occurs for 9 per cent of men who have sex less than once a month.

MEN ON SEX

Half of the 'four-plus times a week' men take advantage of social occasions to indulge in sexual fantasies, and this group also tends to fantasise while watching films or television.

Men who have the most sex seem to be more turned on by social situations than when they're on their own. Fantasising in the bath, for example, holds less of an appeal for the 'four-plus' men. The men most likely to equate the bathroom with sexy thoughts are those who have sex once a fortnight or less than once a month.

OBJECTS OF FANTASY

So far as these are concerned, men tend to be fairly realistic: they prefer to invite people they know into their imaginations rather than film stars.

WHO'S YOUR FANTASY?

Someone not with you at the time	48%
Someone you know vaguely	36%
One of your friends	35%
Someone at work	27%
A film star	27%
No-one in particular	25%
Someone with you at the time	21%
Someone you've only seen once or twice	20%
A TV star	20%
Sports personality	8%
One of your relatives	4%

Men in the discussion groups confirmed that fantasies work best when it's someone you know. According to a single 27 year old: 'You'd have to know them fairly well to be able to maintain an image of them in your head. It depends on the extent of the fantasy. For masturbation, it would have to be more than just a passing person.'

Almost half the men in our survey tend to fantasise about someone who isn't with them at the time, and these are more likely to be men who aren't in a relationship and those who have very little or no sex. It's interesting that 28 per cent of men having the most sex *and* men who have sex less than once a month tend to fantasise about someone they're with at the time. This suggests a link between the two groups: it could be that both sets of men are equally lascivious, but the most sexually active men have more luck!

Young men and the unemployed are the most likely to have fantasies about someone they know vaguely or have only met once or twice, as are men with occasional relationships or none at all. The young and those without work also tend to have sexy thoughts about their friends. Single men form another group which relies on friends as fantasy material, as do two-timers and men with occasional relationships. Fantasies about work colleagues are particularly prevalent among high-earning men, those in the South of England and men who are currently without a relationship.

Whiling away the hours dreaming about film stars, TV stars or sports personalities does not appeal much to older men. It's much more common for men who left school at 16 and those who lost their virginity late. In the small group discussions, men said they enjoyed looking at women on the small screen, but that they were not generally the stuff of hot and sweaty fantasies.

A quarter of men don't feature anyone in particular in their fantasies. This lack of imagination seems most common among men in their late 30s, married and cohabiting men, men with young children and a third of men who've only had one partner. Men who have the *least* trouble thinking of someone to think about are the unemployed, separated men, two-timers and men who never have sex.

SEX OBJECTS?

To probe the subject further, we gave the men in our sample a list of public figures and asked which they found most attractive. Patsy Kensit came top, though she attracted less than a quarter of men in the sample. One in five respondents – 19 per cent – didn't care for any of them! Men in the groups complained there was no obvious 'long blonde hair' type, and were generally more given to

MEN ON SEX

making disparaging remarks than admiring ones. A couple of comments on the questionnaires also criticised the omission of Julia Roberts, Sherilyn Fenn and any black women.

Patsy Kensit's fans are predominantly young, single men on relatively low wages. However, she might be less than pleased with this assessment by a married 39 year old: 'Patsy Kensit is attractive in a sluttish sort of way. She'd be the media's choice.'

Sharron Davies appeals to those in their late 20s and men with basic education. A quarter of the men having sex more than four times a week say she's their pin-up.

A married 27 year old gave his vote to Gabriella Sabatini: 'I love the Mediterranean look. She's more sort of fit all over, as opposed to Sharron Davies.' Other men joining his approval for the tennis star are likely to be young men, two-timers and men having sex once or twice a month. Nastassia Kinski, however, appeals most to men in their late 20s, those with degrees and men in management who earn over £25k. Only 2 per cent of separated men find her attractive, and the two-timers don't fancy her much either. However, a quarter of men who never have sex are attracted to her.

Felicity Kendal is the choice of the older man. Men over 40 and the highest earners go for her in a big way, and she also has support from the men who lost their virginity late. Similarly, Julie Christie gains support from the older men and those in management positions.

None of the other six women on our list earns more than 5 per cent support from our sample, with Anneka Rice and Paula Yates gaining 5 per cent and 4 per cent respectively. Four per cent of men having sex more than four times a week are attracted to Anita Roddick. Joan Collins may be less pleased to learn that it's men without any relationship at all who are keenest on her! At the bottom of the league, Ruby Wax and Margaret Thatcher attract a few votes from separated men.

Fantasy seems to play a big role for the majority of men, and acts both as a substitute and a spur for sexual activity. But, according to men in the groups, the most satisfying fantasy occurs before they first go to bed with a new partner – when having sex is a fantasy almost bound to come true.

11.

Danger! Men at Play

Do you remember when people were scared of catching herpes? Ten years ago, that was the worst that could happen. Now – as we know – things are different. The Government has tried to scare us with ominous icebergs and stories of the holiday romance from hell. But has the message about AIDS got through – and who takes the scaremongering seriously?

THE CONDOM QUESTION

The most obvious way to assess men's awareness of AIDS is by measuring their use of condoms. The condom – once the butt of endless jokes – has now risen above its furtive origins to become a media star of gigantic proportions. A huge number of column inches have been devoted to prophylactics, and this exposure has only helped them on the road to prominence. Added to the fact that they can be life savers. We'll look at the condom as contraception later, but first, we explore their role as the great protector against AIDS.

Almost half the men in our sample say they definitely would not have sex with a new partner without using a condom, and overall, 71 per cent are in favour of wearing a condom the first time with someone new.

This clear evidence that most men take the threat of AIDS seriously and take positive steps to protect themselves and their partners was backed up by comments made on the questionnaires and in the discussion groups. As a married 32 year old in one of

I WOULD USE A CONDOM FOR SEX WITH A NEW PARTNER

Strongly agree	48%
Tend to agree	23%
Neither	7%
Tend to disagree	7%
Strongly disagree	3%
Don't know	12%

the groups said: 'If I was working away and I chanced upon an encounter, I think that maybe a couple of years ago, I wouldn't have worn one. I wouldn't have sex without one now. I don't know what effect the heat of the moment would have, but you'd have to be very irresponsible to yourself.' Of course, in this kind of situation, there may well be a discrepancy between a man's intentions and his actual behaviour.

A single 30 year old felt that AIDS had influenced the choice of contraception in his eight-month relationship with his girlfriend. 'In our relationship we still use condoms, whereas I can think of other relationships that have gone on this long where, by this stage, she would have gone on the Pill. It was the next stage in the seriousness hierarchy.'

For some men, fear of AIDS has even promoted abstinence: 'I feel sex will never play an important part in anyone's life because of the way it is abused today – especially by youngsters. I am very happy that I have never had sex at all with men or women. In fact I would be scared to for fear of catching AIDS,' says a single man in his early 40s, living in London. This is of course a post-rational justification, as AIDS could not have been a factor for this man until he reached his 30s.

Young men are the keenest to use condoms: 76 per cent say they would at least tend to wear one for sex with a new partner, compared with only 62 per cent of men over 40. All men over the age of 30 are much more likely to say they don't know what they'd do: this could be because they're more likely to be in stable monogamous relationships than men under 24. Other groups who are unlikely to know how they'd react given the chance of sex with a new partner include married men and those who've only had one partner.

The finding that young men are the keenest on using condoms was confirmed in a 1990 survey of over 5,000 men conducted for LRC, the manufacturers of Durex condoms. This research found that the youngest age group – 16-20 year olds – saw the highest increase in condom usage between the summers of 1989 and 1990. In their view, this growth reflected the fact that 43 per cent of sexually active 16-20 year olds in their survey said they'd had sex before the legal age of consent. This compares with 20 per cent of our sample who claimed to have lost their virginity before the age of 16. The growth in condom usage also reflected an increased awareness among young men of the risk of AIDS: the survey found that concern about HIV/AIDS grew substantially between 1989 and 1990.

Although more than two-thirds of men in our sample would not have sex with a new partner without using a condom, a closer look at the figures reveals some more disturbing evidence. As the first table in this chapter showed, 48 per cent of the sample said they strongly agreed they would use a condom for sex with a new partner. Yet this is the case for only 39 per cent of men who've had more than ten partners, and 40 per cent of those having sex more than four times a week. Those who've only had one partner and men who don't have sex at the moment are, on the other hand, more likely than average to say they would use a condom, as the following table shows:

I WOULD DEFINITELY USE A CONDOM FOR SEX WITH A NEW PARTNER	
Men who never have sex	57%
Men who've had one partner	51%
All (average)	48%
Men who have sex at least four times a week	40%
Men who've had more than ten partners	39%

If we take into account those in the two groups of sexual athletes who say they more than likely *wouldn't* use a condom, we see that on balance, it's the men who've had more partners who are least likely to insist on a condom.

MEN ON SEX

The Durex survey also found that the men in their survey who had the highest number of new partners were also the most likely to have unprotected sex. According to that report, it was men in the 18-20 age group who were most likely to have taken that risk. The report states: 'It is probably not surprising that it is the 18-24 age group who are taking the most risks, but the fact that over one in four people aged between 18 and 20 have had unprotected sex with a new partner is very disturbing. This is particularly so when this age group is actually also likely to have a higher number of new partners during the year.'

Separated and single men are more likely than married and cohabiting men to say they wouldn't use a condom. And the two-timers – the men who have twice as much fun with twice as many people – are more likely to say they probably wouldn't use a condom: 21 per cent of two-timing men would tend not to insist on a prophylactic, compared with 10 per cent of all our men.

It's also interesting that men who lost their virginity early and those who enjoyed it a lot the first time are less likely to come out strongly in support of condoms. In Chapter 7 we established that these Early Learners live fast. It seems they live dangerously, too.

A certain lack of concern and denial of risk among the sexually active also came across in the group interviews. A single 19-year-old student admitted: "I should use condoms, perhaps, but I don't. I often think about it, but I feel the women at university – I know it's stupid – but I feel they're safer.'

There were also the traditional complaints that condoms lessen sensitivity: 'You don't want to wear a condom; it's like washing your feet with your socks on,' said a married 43 year old. A single 22 year old from the West Midlands had a more disturbing explanation: 'Whilst on Ecstasy one's sexual drive is extremely heightened to the extent that the risk of contracting a sexual disease does not come into the mind, and amongst the heterosexual populace, it contributes a lot to the spread of HIV.'

THE RISK FACTOR

The Durex survey found that half of those questioned did not think they were at risk of contracting the virus themselves, and a relatively small number of people said they were more careful about the kind of partner they had. Only 34 per cent of men claimed to have changed their behaviour in the light of the AIDS risk, while one in ten men said they had fewer sexual partners as a result. A third of the men and women in this survey thought it was only homosexuals and drug addicts who were really at risk of contracting the disease.

But how great is the risk?

The Department of Health's UK figures for the last quarter of 1991 indicate that heterosexual men should take note of the threat of AIDS. The cumulative total of reported AIDS cases was 5,451 of whom 3,391 have died, while the total number of reported cases of HIV infection was 16,828. In 1991, there were 180 reports in the UK of AIDS in men and women infected through heterosexual sexual intercourse – a 50 per cent increase on the number reported in 1990. According to the then Minister for Health: 'These figures show that although the total number is smaller than other groups, the increase in the heterosexual population is faster than in other groups. Many of these heterosexuals have been infected through sexual contact in other countries where prevalence is high, or with someone who has been to such a country.' On the subject of protection, she had this to say: 'Regardless of where or how the infection is acquired, HIV is established in the UK and can be passed on. HIV infection is preventable. Everyone must learn the lessons on how to protect themselves and others. It is important to know the facts, but it is not enough. People need to put the knowledge into practice. Prevention is the only way.'

We asked Da Choong of the Terrence Higgins Trust if there were any indications of an explosion in the growth of heterosexuals contracting AIDS. 'Early estimates [of heterosexual infection] were overplayed to some degree,' she said. 'Over the last five years, the numbers haven't exploded as was originally estimated. This has made people more sceptical and complacent, and the tabloid press has latched on to this, saying HIV and AIDS only affect drug users and gay men. This continues to be a struggle for health educators to overcome.'

Choong also believes that HIV test results do not reflect an accurate measure of the true numbers of heterosexuals infected with the virus. 'People with HIV stay relatively healthy for a long time. Unless you see yourself as at risk, you probably won't take a test – and heterosexuals generally don't see themselves as at risk.' In her view, the anonymous testing of pregnant women gives a more accurate picture of the heterosexual infection rate. These figures show a steady rise in the number of women infected by heterosexual sex with non-high-risk partners.

MEN ON SEX

HOMO SAPIENS?

The Department of Health figures confirm that, although the fastest growth-rate may be among the heterosexual population, AIDS is still predominantly a problem for specific high-risk groups. Of these, the gay population has probably had the longest time to adjust to the effects of HIV and AIDS. So how different are heterosexual and homosexual attitudes to AIDS as a personal risk? We asked Keith Alcorn, assistant editor of the *National AIDS Manual*, a regularly updated guide to information about AIDS for people working in the field. Whereas we found that men with more partners are the least likely to use a condom with a new partner, his information suggests that gay men hold the opposite view. 'Research has been done by Project Sigma at South Bank Polytechnic, as part of an ongoing study of the sexual behaviour of gay men in this country. This has discovered that the more partners gay men have, the more likely they are to be using condoms. The people most likely *not* to be using condoms were those in relationships, because these are people with one committed partner.' He observed that some gay men were more keen to rely on the perceived 'prophylactic effect' of a relationship rather than actual condoms! 'Other studies have also shown that the only significant predictor of whether somebody is having unsafe sex is their relationship. Men in a relationship were four times more likely to be practising unsafe sex, irrespective of whether they were tested for HIV.'

Alcorn gives a brief history of gay men's reaction to AIDS in this country: 'Four to five years ago, Project Sigma saw people changing their sexual practices quite dramatically. They stopped having anal sex altogether. Now they're doing it again, but with condoms. And far more people are having oral sex now, as the evidence suggests it's not a route of transmission for the virus.'

So gay men have adopted safer sexual practices. But what was their motivation? Alcorn believes the general public has swallowed the myth that homosexual men were scared into action by the spectre of personal tragedy on their doorsteps. 'There's a fallacy about why gay men started using condoms. The belief is that it's because people's friends were dying of AIDS and people were testing positive. That didn't happen. What happened is that people began to receive information through the gay press and community organisations. It was because of the community structure that people changed their behaviour. That's partly why the AIDS figures here are not as bad as they are in the US or France.'

But what are the factors that will persuade heterosexual men to change their sexual behaviour? 'Now, the argument is that straight men won't change till they see their friends affected. But are there the same mediums for educating straight men as for gay men? There are certainly magazines, such as *Esquire*, *The Face* and *i-D*, that have taken the issue seriously. Maybe changing women's behaviour is the key. But given the power imbalance in relationships, it could be a lot more difficult to educate straight men. I've been dubious about the possibility of a heterosexual explosion as the rate of partner change is much lower: gay men do have more partners.' However, he conceded that our findings could suggest certain groups of heterosexual men may be more at risk than he'd previously thought.

Be Prepared!

We asked men in our sample if they were prepared for safe sex and if so, in which circumstances. Seventy-six per cent of men *never* carry condoms around with them. If they are going to a social function without a partner, 7 per cent sometimes take condoms, 2 per cent often do and 1 per cent always take them. Irrespective of where they are going, 5 per cent sometimes take condoms, 4 per cent always do and 3 per cent often take them. One man added that he didn't carry condoms because his girlfriend was on the pill, whereas a single 39 year old living in London commented: 'I carry condoms *respective* of where I am going – i.e. when visiting my partner.'

The young, single, non fathers and those with occasional relationships are the most likely to carry condoms, whereas married men, people with a regular partner, and men over 35 are among the least likely to carry them about. Most married men in the discussion groups felt that the idea of carrying condoms around was fairly irrelevant. However, a few did express the opinion that if they did have the opportunity of extra-marital sex, they'd be irresponsible not to use one.

Young single men were split between those who would use condoms with a new partner (contraceptive purposes are a factor here), and those who thought they should, but didn't. However, whether or not they carried condoms themselves, all the men claimed they would encourage their sons and (most) daughters to have condoms at hand when they were older.

There's evidence to suggest that the men least likely to be

MEN ON SEX

having sex are most likely to be prepared for it! Nine per cent of men without a relationship *always* take condoms out with them, and 25 per cent of these men *sometimes* take condoms when they're going to a social function without a partner. The same applies for 23 per cent of men having sex less than once a month, and 18 per cent of those who are currently sexually inactive.

Asked if they keep condoms at home, 43 per cent said they never do; 30 per cent always do; 17 per cent sometimes do; and 9 per cent often do. Men who always have condoms at home tend to have higher education and higher earnings. Separated men, those in occasional relationships and people who lost their virginity late are also likely candidates. You are most unlikely to find a packet of three in the homes of older men, married men, fathers, two-timers and Northerners. Tying in with previous findings, those who never have sex are much less likely to say they *never* keep condoms at home: only 23 per cent say this, compared with 42 per cent of men having sex more than four times a week.

A single 27 year old in one of the groups explained why he didn't use condoms. 'I've got them at home, but I've never used them. I've only had sex with the one girl – still! Since I broke up with her I've been to bed with a lot more people. Well, I've been to bed with four different people this year already, three of them on the same day. I do think about AIDS and that, but I don't have penetrative sex with the people I go to bed with, although in some cases it's practically a technicality. Not for that reason [i.e. AIDS], but because for a long time I've felt you shouldn't have sex with somebody you don't love.'

'At the moment I feel no need to keep condoms either on my person or in the home. However, if my circumstances changed I would keep condoms in the house or take part in non-penetrative sex,' commented a divorced 27 year old living in the South East.

WOMEN WITH CONDOMS SHOCK

What are men's attitudes towards women who are prepared for safe sex? Thirty-eight per cent say they definitely would *not* be put off a woman if they knew she carried condoms. In all, more than half (56 per cent) say they wouldn't object to a woman if they knew she carried condoms; only 17 per cent would regard it as a turn-off, with the rest indifferent. The men most inclined to run in the opposite direction once they sight a woman with condoms are more likely to be older men, married men and fathers. Those who are least likely to object include the youngest men: 47 per cent of men under 24 strongly believe in women carrying condoms, compared with only 29 per cent of the over 40s.

There are several reasons why men might object to a woman who carries condoms. Firstly, men with more traditional views might not like the idea of a woman taking control of the situation and being prepared for sex, should the occasion arise. Then there are those who quite simply don't like condoms (see our foot-washing example above). Finally, there are the men who don't consider themselves at risk and therefore don't see the need for safe sex.

Some interesting patterns emerge from our survey which suggest in which of these groups various types of men would belong. A fairly low number of men who've only ever had one partner (45 per cent) say they wouldn't be put off by a woman carrying condoms, compared with 62 per cent of those who've had more than ten. The more partners a man has had, the less shocked he's likely to be at the sight of condoms in a woman's bag.

The two-timers also have a relatively low tolerance for condoms. However, their reaction probably results from a denial that they're at risk and a dislike of your average prophylactic, rather than shock.

Men who are in regular relationships are slightly less tolerant than average of the idea of a woman carrying condoms; 52 per cent say it wouldn't put them off her. But those with occasional relationships or none at all are the least concerned. Sixty-four per cent of men with occasional relationships say they don't mind if a woman has a packet of three, along with 71 per cent of men without a relationship. These men obviously don't take the view that nice girls don't carry condoms, and are not likely to stop a condom coming between them and sex.

FIRST-DATE SEX

Asked if they would lose respect for a woman who was prepared to sleep with them on a first date, the men who say they would still respect her are ahead by a slight margin.

Overall, 35 per cent disagree and 31 per cent agree. Older men are much less worried about the issue than younger men: only 26 per cent of men over 40 say they wouldn't respect a

I WOULDN'T RESPECT A WOMAN WHO WAS PREPARED TO SLEEP WITH ME ON A FIRST DATE

Strongly agree	15%
Tend to agree	16%
Neither	24%
Tend to disagree	17%
Strongly disagree	18%
Don't know	10%

woman in the morning, compared with 37 per cent of those under 24. This could be evidence of younger men leading a swing back to old-fashioned morality, in the light of their higher consciousness of the AIDS threat.

This attitude is backed up by a single 26 year old from the East Midlands: 'Today, I feel that I have much more respect for women than I did in my late teens and early 20s. Therefore this has had a marked influence on my attitude to sex. But although I no longer go out thinking of the possibility of a one-night stand, it would be hypocritical of me to claim that I would be repelled by the idea. Also, like many other people I am always mindful of the consequences of AIDS. Finally, today, I consider the idea of a relationship to be much more appealing than any form of casual sex.'

Agony aunt Claire Rayner agrees that AIDS could be behind this change of outlook, but doesn't think it will last forever: 'The volume of sexual activity has always been a cyclical thing. In the late 18th century, men and women were sexing and whoring all the time – the women dressed in damp muslin to show their breasts and the shadow of their pubic hair. Then came the sexual repression of the mid-Victoria era, then the Naughty Nineties and so on – up and down – until free love in the Sixties. Now we are almost at the top of a right wing swing back to primness and propriety. AIDS has put an end to the friendly fuck so there is less penetrative sex and more petting coming back; half the headache and no risk. But come the end of the century, I think there will be another revolution. We'll be back to the naughtiness again.'

As we've seen before, the men least likely to get into the situation of having sex with someone new are most likely not to know how they'd react. Thirteen per cent of married men, 14 per cent of the cohabitors and 17 per cent of men who've only had one partner say they don't know whether or not they'd respect a woman who would sleep with them on a first date.

Men who've only had one partner are among the most likely to think badly of a woman who would be willing to have sex on the first date, as are 43 per cent of men who never have sex. It's also significant that those who lost their virginity late and hardly enjoyed the experience at all are more likely to disapprove strongly of this idea. These findings indicate a puritanical streak in the two groups of men who are sexually inactive and late starters.

The following table shows the differences in men's opinions according to their levels of sexual experience and activity.

I WOULDN'T RESPECT A WOMAN WHO WAS PREPARED TO SLEEP WITH ME ON THE FIRST DATE

	AGREE	DISAGREE
Average	31%	35%
Men who've had one partner	37%	27%
Men who've had more than ten partners	27%	46%
Men who never have sex	43%	27%
Men who have sex at least four times a week	33%	36%

It doesn't come as a surprise that the men who've had most partners are the keenest on the idea of a woman who'll have sex with them straightaway. But it's interesting that men who have the most sex have a more restrained view.

ZERO POP

'Zero Pop' would make a great name for a condom, but is in fact the name of a pressure group pushing for zero population growth.

MEN ON SEX

And so to the issue of contraception. The condom is the most popular method for the men in our survey, used by 41 per cent of those who have sex these days. Condom use peaks in the South and is most popular with the young.

More than 10 per cent of those who are currently active sexually have had a vasectomy, and this is much more popular among the group of men over 40, those who are married and the two-timers. The partners of 31 per cent use the pill – and this is most popular for those in their late 20s and the cohabitors. Such devices as the coil and diaphragm appear to have lost whatever popularity they once enjoyed, with 3 and 2 per cent respectively. Only 1 per cent use abstinence to reduce the risk of unwanted fatherhood. However, 8 per cent favour the other non-technical approach – withdrawal – which is particularly popular with men who've had more than ten partners.

MEN WHO USE CONDOMS FOR CONTRACEPTION/PROTECTION

AGE	
18-24	62%
25-29	43%
30-34	41%
35-39	29%
40-45	22%

Condoms are widely used by singles, non-fathers, the One-Woman Men and men who aren't having much sex at the moment (i.e. less than once a month). However, those with a lot of sexual experience are less keen on condoms.

Our survey confirms the finding in the Durex report that the condom is the most popular form of contraception in Britain. Sales of condoms have risen dramatically during the last decade, from 109 million condoms in 1983 to 148 million in 1991. The reasons for this growth include increasing concern about HIV and AIDS, government promotion of condoms, a reaction against methods of contraception such as the Pill, and the fact that condoms are now more widely available and more widely promoted. The Durex survey confirms that Londoners are keener on condoms than men elsewhere in Britain: in their survey, 35 per cent of men in London use condoms, compared with 22 per cent of those in Yorkshire, and 25 per cent of Scots.

Over two-thirds of men in our survey have taken on board the idea that sex can be bad for your health, and are prepared to use condoms to protect themselves. And just over half of them would not be shocked by a woman who carried condoms, although they are divided as to whether they would respect someone who'd have sex on a first date. The most alarming side of men at play is the number who've had more than ten partners who probably wouldn't use a condom for sex with a new partner. There may not be a heterosexual explosion of AIDS yet, but a significant minority ignoring the risk could change all that.

FIRST RESPONSE PROFILE

Name:	John
Age:	28
Occupation:	Journalist
Lives:	South East
Sexuality:	Heterosexual
Relationship:	Cohabiting
Virginity loss:	14, enjoyable experience
Sexual activity	More than 4 times a week? – absolutely not!

Foreword

I don't like the phrase 'Sexual Athletes' because my notion of an athlete is someone who is quite dedicated and responsible,

MEN ON SEX — whereas in this research it shows that this category are among the most irresponsible of men. It seems to me like a glamorous endorsement of something that might not be glamorous at all. I've heard government spokespeople classify anyone who's had sex with more than six partners as promiscuous. That makes me a promiscuous sexual athlete – and I resent that labelling. 'Highly sexually active' would be more appropriate.

Would You Use a Condom for Sex with a New Partner?

I would definitely use a condom with a new partner – in fact, I'd put myself in the 'Strongly Agree' category. The reason is, not too long ago I had an affair with someone and didn't use a condom and I thought, 'If I'm someone aware of the issues and the risks and I haven't changed my behaviour, then there can't be any hope for the rest of us.' One of the things that came out of that experience was I began doing some work for an AIDS organisation as a volunteer, so have contact with someone who has AIDS. I think it's very unlikely that I would have unprotected sex now.

I'd love to know the thinking of the people who came into the 'Strongly Disagree' category. I think they're probably being conned into thinking that they're in a low-risk group when the point is that low-risk groups don't exist – there are just lower-risk forms of behaviour. Unprotected penetrative sex and exchange of body fluids with a new partner is always a high-risk activity. No matter what you may think you know about another person's behaviour and sexual history, there is no way you can know anything about their previous partner's sexual behaviour and history. The whole thing makes me angry when I think that if gay people can understand, then why can't straight people?

Full Circle

In terms of using condoms generally, I'm sure my own experience is common to many men of my age – which is that when I first had sex, condoms were the only form of contraception available. Then as we grew older, our girlfriends took control of their own contraception and started to use the Pill or the cap. Now, I know very few women who are still on the Pill. Everyone seems to have come back to condoms – where we started.

Sexual Etiquette

It doesn't surprise me that the people who have the most partners are the least likely to insist on using a condom, because I suppose part of the problem is, the first time you sleep with someone is the worst time to have to negotiate such difficult issues. You've therefore got a lot more 'first times' to negotiate. Also, the issue of contraception immediately raises the issue of both health and pregnancy, and if you want to get someone into bed those are the last things you want to raise! So I see a sort of 'seducer's logic' to the whole thing.

When people use references like eating sweets with the wrapper on, washing feet with socks on, etc., what they're really saying is that sexual pleasure is more important than killing your partner – not a very justifiable position. I do agree, and know from experience, that any form of contraception can feel like a barrier between you and your partner. But surely you just have to waive that pleasure against the risk. The final statistics about people not believing they are at risk from HIV are just depressing, really.

I agree that the most alarming side of men at play is men with most partners who wouldn't use a condom for sex with a new partner. Common sense tells you that those men probably aren't going to change, therefore what has to happen is that women have to stop sleeping with them. There's no other way – women have to protect themselves from these men.

Lots of women probably wouldn't miss all that penetrative sex, anyway! I think that's the big secret, actually. The explosive thing about this whole issue is that it's the men who miss the humping most! And now women have got a good argument for saying no!

The good thing about the discussion about sexual behaviour that's been triggered by HIV and AIDS is that people have had to confront what they actually do in their sexual behaviour. And it's demonstrated real responsibility on the part of the gay community and the fact that we should end up in a world where people can do what they like with who they like, as long as they wear a condom.

Survival Tactics

I welcome the fact that trendy men's magazines have all done condom issues. I remember the *i-D* issue in particular, where they gave away free condoms and had lots of celebrity interviews. One of the best things they did was have positive profiles of people who were HIV, because as well as stopping people getting the illness you have to accept the people who do have it. It seems as though a lot of the anxiety we have about death, we focus on a particular illness. In the early 70s, it was cancer. It was more frightening and taboo than even death itself, and that is sort of what has happened to AIDS now – it's the most frightening way of dying. But it's not really, it's just one of the many. So those articles help people to live with it, survive it.

Carrying Condoms

I always carry condoms and know a lot of people who work in the AIDS industry who carry condoms as a mark of being perceived correct. I don't think that's any bad thing. I think you'd have to be fairly Neanderthal to object to women carrying condoms. The same people who object to women carrying condoms probably wouldn't even raise an eyebrow if the woman were on the Pill and that's really just because the Pill is invisible. So it's nothing more than a kind of squeamishness, really. I suppose it's also about giving women control over men's bodies, which – I guess – is threatening. But if you're worried about that you're probably not very good in bed anyway!

I think if you think you're ever going to have an affair, then you know that you're going to have to use condoms. If you don't and you have an affair – that means afterwards, you may have to start using condoms to protect your partner. There are two things: one, you should start as you mean to go on; and two, we've got to break the connection between condoms and infidelity. I know a lot of women have a lot of problems about suddenly insisting on their partners using condoms because they suspect their partners are being unfaithful – when in actual fact, what they're saying is 'I'm protecting myself because I don't trust *you!*' It's no use telling the women to go home and use condoms because it's practically impossible to get men to do things you want them to do. So men have to lead from the front, really. Whereas in gay relationships the power relationship is much more even. In heterosexual couples the obligation is more on the man to do the right thing. Women can't make men use condoms.

First-date Sex

Suspecting a woman who's prepared to sleep with me on a first date seems such a daft thing to me. It implies that phrase about 'respecting a woman' which comes from a staid vocabulary of courtship that hasn't got anything to do with my life – along with 'making an honest woman of her'. Quite laughable really. It's just male hypocrisy, isn't it? Just stupid. I might not respect her if she wasn't prepared to use a condom or was embarrassed to use one – that seems to me more important. Because if you didn't use a condom with me, why should I imagine that you did with the last person you slept with?

New-age Dawns

I'm very glad that Claire Rayner thinks we're going back to naughtiness, because I think men of my age had the freedom of the Pill snatched away from us when we suddenly realised it was damaging women's health. Then you saw promiscuity made far more difficult with the advent of AIDS. Then we had to get used to wearing condoms again, like we did when we were teenagers – and at the same time we had to listen to people rhapsodising about the '60s! So I'm looking forward to a big safe sex revival in the year 2000, along with a cure for AIDS!

12.

Danger! Men at Work

We've already seen that job satisfaction is the top priority for half the men in our sample. The survey also shows that the majority of our men spend more than eight hours a day at work. Here's a run-down of men's work timetables.

NUMBER OF HOURS WORKED PER WEEK	
1-7 hours	1%
8-29 hours	5%
30-39 hours	18%
40-49 hours	41%
50-59 hours	17%
60-69 hours	7%
70 hours	2%
Not stated	9%

If you accept the suggestion that a man working an average of ten hours a day, five days a week, is verging on workaholism, that puts over a quarter of our men in this category. The men most likely to do so are those over 35, men who earn more than £25k, those in higher employment, married men and men who've had more than ten partners.

Given that men place such importance in their work and devote so much time to it, we wanted to find out how they interact with women in the workplace – on both a professional and personal level.

The Career Ladder

We delved into the emotive areas of women at work and positive discrimination. Just over a quarter of men think women have a better chance of getting on in their careers than men – a surprisingly high figure. This table shows men's views.

WOMEN HAVE MORE CHANCE OF CAREER PROGRESSION THAN MEN	
Strongly agree	6%
Tend to agree	21%
Neither	24%
Tend to disagree	34%
Strongly disagree	13%
Don't know	3%

In the group discussions, men generally paid lip service to the notion that it's still a man's world, and that women sometimes experience discrimination at work. A married 35-year-old teacher said: 'I've certainly been in the position where a woman has been passed over. It's been, look at her age, recently married. She'll be off having children and we'll be back where we started.'

A single 22 year old living in Scotland has strong feelings on how women should operate to further their careers: 'In an opportunity sense, men have more of a deal than women in promotion, salary and conditions. But I would also say women should stop moaning and join the bandwagon in the opportunity stakes. As they say, "If you don't go for it, you don't get it." I know this from experience with women who didn't moan and now they are rather well placed in companies.'

Labour MP Ken Livingstone is in no doubt that women are

MEN ON SEX

put at a disadvantage at work: 'I can't think of a single frontline profession in Britain where there isn't discrimination. It's systematic and institutionalised throughout British society. Women can't do more, short of knee-capping men on the way to meetings.' And in his view, these restrictions are particularly relevant in the world of politics: 'The House of Commons is a very hostile environment for women. Labour has only 10 per cent women MPs, Tories 5 per cent. There's a general fear that women are more radical and will challenge their privileges. The problem is the party machines: they are very racist, very sexist.'

His attitude is in stark contrast to that of Conservative MP Sir Teddy Taylor: 'I certainly don't think we are blocking women in any way in the House of Commons. We're very polite to them. I am *always* polite to them. There's no prejudice against women in general. There is prejudice against particular women MPs because they have nasty characters. As far as sexism in the country is concerned, it's illegal. You're not allowed to do that now.'

Men in higher forms of employment (and hence presumably those in the best position to judge women's advancement into the higher echelons in the workplace) are more likely than the rest to feel women do have a better chance of promotion than men. However, 52 per cent of this group also disagree that this is true.

Forty-eight per cent of the unemployed agree women have a better chance to get on than men. This may be due to their youth and more progressive ideas, or it could be sour grapes. Men over 40 are more likely to feel women don't have an advantage, along with men with higher education, those earning over £25k, and men who've had more than ten partners.

Most men are fairly cool towards the idea of positive discrimination in favour of women. Thirty per cent don't have an opinion about it, 20 per cent think it's a good idea, while 44 per cent are not in favour. Those who've only had one partner are less likely to agree with the idea than those who've had the most partners. Meanwhile, two-timers think it's a terrible notion. As does Sir Teddy Taylor, who considers any form of positive discrimination to be a backward step: 'There is nothing one can realistically do to change things without fiddling the system, and that never works. The women wouldn't be the same calibre, and they wouldn't have the same standing. It would undermine the things that are important about Britain, like equal opportunities. And women *do* have equal opportunities.'

Exactly half the men in our sample believe that there are equal opportunities for men and women where they work. Among the rest, 10 per cent say there is no policy one way or another, 24 per cent say there aren't equal opportunities, and 17 per cent don't know. The youngest group of men under 24 are the least likely to agree: only 44 per cent say men and women have an equal opportunity to progress, compared with 53 per cent of older men. In terms of income, it's interesting that only 15 per cent of those earning over £25k are convinced there's a policy of equality where they work (however, 32 per cent tend to agree this is the case). Men who have sex at least four times a week are particularly likely to agree that there are equal opportunities.

MALE OR FEMALE BOSS?

But what about relationships at work with those in authority? Over half the men in our survey don't mind whether they have a male or female boss.

WHO'S THE BEST?	
Man	39%
Woman	4%
No difference	52%
Don't know	6%

However, if a man does prefer to work for another man, it doesn't necessarily mean he hates women, as a single 30 year old from London explained: 'By and large most women are affected by periods and body imbalances. Women have strong mood swings and at times are prone to unnecessary chit-chat (fact).' This was not an isolated opinion, and this view is still frequently put forward as a reason for keeping women out of the boardroom.

Married men are less happy than cohabiting, separated or single men to take orders from a woman. Only 1 per cent of them say they'd prefer a female boss, compared with 8 per cent of single men. The same holds true for men in regular relationships – they're less likely than men with occasional or no relationships to want a woman in command. This suggests that married men and

MEN ON SEX

those in steady relationships tend towards a more traditional view of the sexes.

Men who like the idea of a female boss are more likely to be the young; 9 per cent of men under 24 would prefer a woman boss. However, this idea only appeals to 1 per cent of men over 40. Many more of the older men and higher earners prefer to stick to the traditional arrangement in which they have a male boss.

IS THERE AN OFFICE GROPER?

Sexual harassment is a question of manipulation – an abuse of power – with the person in authority taking advantage of their position. Someone working in the post-room is highly unlikely to pinch the financial director's bottom – male or female – but reverse the positions and you have a much more plausible scenario. We asked men in our sample whether sexual harassment of women by men is a problem where they work. Bear in mind that in order to notice it and think it a problem, men have to be aware of the issue in the first place.

SEXUAL HARASSMENT OF WOMEN BY MEN IS A PROBLEM WHERE I WORK	
Strongly agree	3%
Tend to agree	7%
Neither	11%
Tend to disagree	26%
Strongly disagree	35%
Don't know	19%

Overall, 10 per cent say sexual harassment is a problem, while 61 per cent say it isn't. The groups particularly likely to deny strongly that it's a problem include men in their late 20s, those in their early 40s, men in upper management positions, separated men, and those who've had more than ten partners. Others who come into this category are those who have sex at least four times a week, and those who rarely have sex. However, men in their early 30s tend to agree that sexual harassment does occur in their workplace. There's an interesting correlation here with sexual activity. The tendency to agree that sexual harassment is a problem increases with the amount of sexual activity a man has: only 3 per cent of those who never have sex say it's a problem, compared with 11 per cent of men who have sex at least four times a week.

Defining what constitutes harassment is part of the problem. There's often a difference in perception: what a man may see as a friendly squeeze on the arm, a woman may experience as an invasion of her space. Behaviour which is definitely considered to be harassment includes: sexual aggression, sexual propositions, pinching and grabbing. Other sorts of conduct which are also generally agreed to be harassment are: displays of pornographic material, touching or patting, spreading rumours about a person's private life, and continuing to ask women out on dates despite refusal. Suggestive looks at someone's body come into a category that many people are more reluctant to define as harassment, as do questioning or bantering about a person's private life and regular sexual remarks or jokes. Activities least likely to be interpreted as sexual harassment are: others openly discussing their own sexual activities, kissing on the cheek when meeting or parting, and eyeing women up and down.

In 1991, Alfred Marks conducted a survey into attitudes about sexual harassment, which analysed the experiences of 546 temporary clerical/secretarial staff, 82 per cent of whom were female. The great majority of these people (61 per cent) had experience of sexual harassment by the opposite sex, which had taken place on average four times. Compared with these predominantly female respondents, men in our sample are significantly less convinced that sexual harassment is a problem in the workplace. This either means that these men work in much more enlightened circumstances than the people in the Alfred Marks survey, or that sexual harassment simply doesn't come to their attention.

The offender tended to be a colleague or someone at the same level for 46 per cent of the sample, a senior member of staff for 43 per cent, or the immediate boss for 34 per cent. It was mainly seen as a problem involving senior males harassing junior females. The most common reaction for victims was to laugh off the situation, remain cool and uninterested or pretend not to notice. It was much less common for people to make an emphatic verbal reaction or to reject the offender physically. In the past, almost half the victims of sexual harassment did not report the incident or make any complaint. However, 60 per cent thought that, in case of a future incident, they would tell the offender to stop.

In general, people taking part in the survey felt that the reason why so few incidents were reported is that sexual harassment is so hard to define. There was also a strong feeling that the issue should be taken more seriously, and that tougher laws or punishments are needed to combat the problem. Many people were restrained from reporting incidents of sexual harassment by the belief that the organisation would not take any positive action, and it was found that there was a formal written grievance procedure in only 8 per cent of cases.

WORKING RELATIONS

From harassment issues, we moved to the personal, and asked men about the relationships they have with female colleagues.

THERE ARE WOMEN AT WORK I REGARD AS MY FRIENDS

Strongly agree	23%
Tend to agree	36%
Neither	14%
Tend to disagree	5%
Strongly disagree	4%
Don't know	17%

Fifty-nine per cent say they have women friends at work. Men in the 25-35 age group are the most likely to agree with the statement, as are those who are more educated, men in the middle income bracket (£15-25k), those in intermediate managerial posts, separated men and those with occasional relationships or none at all. Female friends at work are most important, however, for the men having very little or no sex. Two-thirds of these men consider some of their women colleagues as friends, as do most of the sexually inactive group.

Married men are less likely to have women friends at work, as are those who've only had one partner and two-timers. Forty-three per cent of men who've only had one partner have a tendency to consider women at work as friends, but − of those with sexual experience − they are the least likely to say female colleagues are definitely counted among their friends.

SEX AT WORK

As we've already established, 35 per cent of men in our sample feel most masculine when they're at work. And 32 per cent fantasise about sex during their working day. So it comes as no surprise that more than half our men are attracted to women at their workplace.

THERE ARE WOMEN AT WORK I FIND SEXUALLY ATTRACTIVE	
Strongly agree	22%
Tend to agree	31%
Neither	9%
Tend to disagree	10%
Strongly disagree	10%
Don't know	18%

It's men over 40 who are most likely to be attracted to female colleagues, while younger men are particularly likely to say they don't know how they feel about women at work. Other men who are likely to be attracted to female colleagues include men who were educated beyond the age of 16, those earning over £15k, men in managerial positions, separated men, those whose children are aged ten or above and men without a relationship.

The least likely to say they feel strongly attracted to women at work are men who are attached − the married and cohabiting men in our sample. However, many of these men say they *tend* to agree there are women at work they find attractive. There is a similar pattern for sexual experience. One-Woman Men are much less

MEN ON SEX

likely than those who've had more than ten partners to say they are strongly attracted to someone at work, but many more say they tend to find women at work attractive. One-Woman Men are just that: they have the least need of all our sample for flirtatious or platonic relationships at work.

However, different rules apply according to sexual activity. It's men who have the least sex who are the most likely to have sex on their mind at work: around a third of these men strongly agree there are women at work they find sexually attractive. This finding confirms the suggestion that this group of men, although sexually inactive in deed, have not stopped thinking about sex.

A further survey by Alfred Marks explored the issue of relationships at work, to find out how common they are and what effect they have on work performance, colleagues and the people involved. Carried out in December 1991, the research analysed responses from 479 temporary staff and permanent job applicants. The results confirmed that most of the people in this survey (58 per cent) had experienced at least one relationship at work. In addition, 68 per cent of the sample had been in a work situation where other colleagues were having a relationship. A surprisingly high number – 51 per cent – of all these relationships led to marriage or the two people living together. For most people, the relationship started through contact made during working hours. However, just over a quarter of people were brought together at the office Christmas party.

In this survey, most people did not think that having a relationship in the workplace had an adverse effect on the work of those involved or the people around them. According to people having relationships at work, there was little disapproval from senior members of staff. However, people in a work situation where colleagues are having an affair were more likely to say that bosses did take slight exception. Around a third opted for a clandestine affair: 32 per cent of people who'd had an affair at work chose to keep it secret, while another 27 per cent only told close friends. Just 1 per cent decided the best thing to do was to act openly. When asked what action they thought organisations should take over office affairs, two-thirds of respondents said they should simply ignore the situation, and 13 per cent said affairs in the office should be discouraged. This contrasts with the 5 per cent who thought they should be encouraged instead.

Interestingly, most people (57 per cent) who experienced a romantic relationship at work were involved with a colleague of the same status. This throws a different light on our finding that it's men in managerial positions who are most likely to be sexually attracted to someone at work. Given the relatively low numbers of women in management, this finding suggests that although senior members of staff may find women at work attractive, women are more likely to have an affair with their peers.

But what happens when the woman's your manager? A 26 year old who fell in love with his boss found that the relationship caused mirth rather than raised eyebrows: 'I'd always go out with someone who is intellectually my equal or superior. In some ways, it was harder for her, being senior to me. But she wasn't so senior it caused a stir. It was just a cause for comment – the main reaction was amusement.' He feels part of the attraction of their 'working relationship' was an understanding of the particular practices of one organisation: 'In our profession, we come under serious pressure and often have to work long hours. People outside don't understand. It helps to have a common knowledge of the environment you work in.' But he was also wary of becoming involved just because the situation presented itself. 'At the start, we had to question ourselves and ask, "Are we just going out with each other because we do the same job, being sucked along in the flow, and looking for someone to talk shop to?"' The couple have now been going out for two and a half years, and are engaged, but he doesn't think their work affair is typical: 'With most people here being in their 20s, most relationships don't last more than a few months.' They have had to develop tactics so that their relationship doesn't interfere with their everyday work roles: 'Increasingly, we've tended to steer clear of each other at work, make it fairly arm's length. We're quite an independent couple, which probably helped.'

This is one example of an office affair leading to marriage. But when one half of the couple is already married different rules apply. A 27 year old from the East Midlands explains the situation which led to his divorce: 'I was working with this girl in the office. We worked very closely together on a project for nine months, spending a lot of time together – a lot of overtime etc. It got to the point where I was spending as much time with her as I was with my wife.' There were a lot of pressures on the relationship with his wife at the time: 'We were planning to go round the world, and had an old house which needed decorating so we could rent it out; that was all down to me. I'd just smashed the car up in France, which put us back another £1,000. Then I was on a management course in the evenings, which took up two evenings a week, two evenings working and one day at the weekend.'

He also feels that his own lack of sexual experience was a factor which encouraged him to start the affair: 'I was married at 25, and was very young and inexperienced. My wife was my first real girlfriend. My wife had had a number of partners before and I hadn't. If I'd had different partners before, it would have been less likely to have happened.' He was horrified at the speed of events, having ruled out a secret affair: 'There was no subterfuge, no clandestine romance – I'm hopeless at that. I told my wife about it. And within a month, I was out. I hadn't appreciated the consequences of telling my wife – that things would fall apart that quickly, come clattering round my earholes. And she was devastated.'

The new relationship lasted for a year, until it came to decision time and he decided to stop and think what he was doing. Now he says: 'I think about things before I do them these days. There isn't anybody who's benefited from it; it costs a bomb to get divorced these days. It must have been awful for my wife – she doesn't deserve the hurt. And she still means an awful lot to me.'

Men in our sample may not think that much grabbing and pinching of women goes on where they work, but half feel a sexual undercurrent running through some of their work relationships. The fact that most men don't see sexual harassment as a problem is graphically contrasted with the experiences of female employees. In the same way, equal opportunities are likely to be less of an issue for men than for women. In an increasingly complex work environment, men and women have to negotiate potentially explosive situations in order to work together. The evidence in our survey suggests that men, at least, manage to define boundaries and juggle work and play, most of the time. But as our last example shows, the man who plays with fire should wear asbestos trousers.

FIRST RESPONSE PROFILE

Name:	Tony
Age:	25
Occupation:	Editor
Lives:	South East
Education:	'O', 'A' levels, degree
Sexuality:	Heterosexual
Relationship:	None
Virginity loss:	16, enjoyed the experience a lot
Hours worked per week:	Over 70

The Equaliser

People's reactions to this subject will depend on their age group. We do have equal opportunities where I work, but there is still a long way to go. The department I work in is predominantly controlled by men in their 50s, and upwards of two-thirds of the people who work there are men. They talk about being approachable, but are not used to equal opportunities, and the situation is probably less than fair. Things are changing, now, with younger management coming through. There's a definite policy of equal opportunities, and a new head of department in his 30s is introducing several new policies specifically for women.

Grabbing Attention

As regards attitudes, you'd probably get a better idea by asking women. I haven't noticed it, but female friends have complained to me about it. It's also a question of how you define sexual harassment. It happens mostly with a particular age group –

MEN
ON
SEX

usually men in their 50s. There's nothing extreme – it's usually verbal comments made unthinkingly. The men who perpetrate it often don't notice the offence they're going to cause, and they probably wouldn't want to cause offence. The women dislike it intensely. Unlike the people mentioned in the survey, my friends actually say something. It's very different for women in a junior situation, but most of the women I work with are very strong characters – highly educated and confident.

I have seen sexual harassment of a man by a dominant woman. It was just physical stuff – hands on legs etc. She did it to establish dominance.

Working Relations

I totally disagree with the idea that it's just men who have sex on their mind at work. It's just the same for women. Men want emotional connection as much as women, and not just physical release. I've had two relationships at work and both were very enjoyable. They lasted for six months each. It's mainly a question of geography – we were working on the same floor. We didn't see each other the whole time. I didn't keep it secret, but wouldn't have wanted people to have any knowledge of them. I work 12-14 hours a day in pressured situations, and people tend to gossip about everything, especially relationships. Relationships go down the grapevine faster than just about anything else! They don't talk about you if you're in the room, but if you're not in the room, you're fair game.

I dislike the way it's implied that men's behaviour is mildly bestial; women do it too. There are so many articles which bash men over the head, accusing men of being insensitive, but there are a lot of men who lack confidence out there as well. At the harassment level, the majority is male to female. But the sexual undercurrent at work definitely works both ways.

I also disagree with the idea that women friends are most important to men without a relationship. There are a lot of men and women out of relationships at the moment. I've got a great deal of female friends at work – it's a very positive situation.

Positive Thinking

There is some positive discrimination – it exists and is a source of irritation to some men when they see women getting perks. But men have to look at the advantages they've had. Over the years, obviously, men have benefited from being male and in certain positions of power. And now it's time the balance changed. They don't see it in those terms, though, and I'm sure they're threatened. I experienced it recently when a job was available and a female candidate was given a place on a training programme. In my opinion, she was given the position because she was a woman. But I don't object to that.

Who's the Best Boss?

I've experienced both male and female bosses and I don't mind either as long as they know what they're doing. But the older men probably wouldn't take too well to a female boss. As for different male and female management styles, I'm tempted to say women are better communicators. But it all depends on the individual person. Women have often had to placate men in relationships, so they're used to that role. That was certainly the case in my family, with my mother placating my father when he was in one of his moods. It was only because he was inarticulate and unable to cope with his feelings.

In my own experience, male and female bosses have usually been quite equal. The sad thing is that in my workplace, it's a shark pool – to compete and succeed is everything. It leads both men and women to behave in a way they probably wouldn't otherwise. I do see women being pushy and aggressive – unfortunately behaving like some of the men. This is only certain individuals, though. They feel the need to compete and adopt the male way – the way they see of progressing. There are the odd one or two who are extremely professional – more balanced and better at communicating. If they want something done, they realise it's better to ask nicely than attempt to bully people.

> MEN ON SEX

13.

And Then There Were Three

The New Man may take naturally to nappies, but there are many fathers who never will, and some who would happily leave the responsibility of child-raising to someone else. Do men embrace the changes that children inevitably bring, or run away from them? We asked the men in our survey about women's and men's involvement in childcare and the role that work plays.

WHO'S LEFT HOLDING THE BABY?

First of all we asked what they thought of the statement that women with pre-school-age children should not go out to work, but should stay at home to look after them. Here are their replies.

WOMEN WITH YOUNG CHILDREN SHOULD STAY AT HOME	
Strongly agree	11%
Tend to agree	26%
Neither	20%
Tend to disagree	23%
Strongly disagree	17%
Don't know	3%

Men are more or less equally divided on this question: overall, 37 per cent think women should stay at home, while 40 per cent disagree. The evidence suggests that young men have more progressive ideas than the oldest men in our sample. Men over 40 are more likely than younger men to be in favour of women staying at home with young children. Others strongly in favour include men with basic education and those who are separated. Fathers are more likely than non fathers to say they *tend* to agree, and the older their children, the more men say this – which is presumably a reflection of their age. Other men who fall into this camp are those earning over £25k, the two-timers and those who lost their virginity late.

A 22 year old cohabiting in the North West told of his experience as a single parent: 'I was left with my baby boy when he was three months old and was a single parent for 15 months. During this time I realised that women are far better with children than men. I think women should not let go of their own value as mothers and housewives.'

Married men are fairly evenly divided in their opinion, with 43 per cent in favour of women looking after pre-school-age children, and 39 per cent against. But in the discussion groups, married men tended to have very traditional views, and most thought that women should stop work when they have children. 'Personally, if you have children, I think it's wrong to then hand them over to a child-minder – I think you shouldn't have them,' said a married 31 year old. Some justified their opinion on the basis of practicalities: 'People that work for me have awful problems fitting their work round their family, because the wife works full time, and if the kid's sick for four days, she has two days, and he has two days,' said a married 32 year old. 'I think I'm very lucky to have a non-working wife.'

In some cases, these attitudes were also bolstered by a sense of pride, with men happy to say their wives didn't need to work. In addition, there was a general conviction that women don't really *want* to work, either. A married 32 year old thought that roles in his house were sensibly divided: 'We're very lucky. I don't wash or dust – she likes to do that sort of thing. I like to work – I couldn't think about not working. So it works well.'

However, some of the younger, single men had a more progressive stance on the issue of childcare. 'I think it's important for a woman to have her own career,' according to a single 29 year old. 'And even when they've had children, from the woman's point of view it's probably better to go back to work. It must be horrendous to have some squalling brat hanging round you all day. Let the child-minder take all the hassle.' For the youngest men, the question of who should look after children was almost too distant to contemplate. 'It's such a big issue, kids and things. I don't even think about it,' said a single 19 year old. 'There's no way I'm having kids for a long time. But I suppose I wouldn't want them with a minder.'

The men who generally think women should work rather than stay at home with their children are likely to be under 35, non fathers and those who have children under the age of nine. Men without a relationship and those who never have sex also tend towards the opposite view.

Those who *strongly* believe a woman's place is at work rather than in the home include men with higher education and those living with children under the age of four, among others.

THE ABSENT FATHER

We wanted to know whether men in our survey thought men should be more involved in caring for their children. Their replies indicated a certain level of guilt.

MEN DON'T DO ENOUGH TO LOOK AFTER THEIR CHILDREN

Strongly agree	8%
Tend to agree	44%
Neither	24%
Tend to disagree	14%
Strongly disagree	4%
Don't know	6%

Men over 35 are more likely than average to say they strongly agree that men could do more to look after their children, as are separated men, those who've had more than ten partners and men who lost their virginity early. The tendency to feel men don't do enough to look after their children is higher for men in their late

30s, and those with a higher level of education. Two-thirds of two-timers come into this category, as do half the married men and fathers. Men with more than ten partners are also much more likely to think men could do more than those who've only had one partner.

A higher than average proportion of separated men strongly disagree that men should do more, as do more of those who never have sex at the moment.

Forty-six per cent of men in our sample *tend* to say that pressure at work is the reason why men don't get enough time with their children. Nineteen per cent are convinced this is the case, 18 per cent don't have an opinion, 8 per cent tend to disagree, 2 per cent strongly disagree and 6 per cent don't know whether work is the obstacle. In the group discussions, there was some agreement that men would like to spend more time with their children, but that work doesn't allow it. However, some believed that when they *did* see them, at least it was 'quality time'. According to a married 38 year old: 'I suppose I feel I would spend more time with my children if I didn't have competing pressures from work. But then again, the time I do spend with them I try to make valuable time.'

The tendency to agree that work gets in the way is greatest for more educated men, those earning over £25k and married men. Strong feelings that men would see more of their children with less pressure at work are expressed by those in their 30s, men who earn most and those with better jobs.

Men who *tend* to disagree are likely to be young – under 24 – with occasional relationships or none and those having sex less than once a month.

IS THERE SEX AFTER CHILDREN?

We asked the 321 fathers in our survey what effect the birth of their first child had on their sex life. Forty-two per cent said it stayed about the same; it deteriorated for 36 per cent; improved for 14 per cent; 7 per cent can't remember; and 1 per cent either didn't know or weren't around after the birth.

A few married men in the discussion groups said that their sex lives worsened after they had children in the sense that they no longer had as much time for sex. They acknowledged that their wives probably felt the same way, too. A married 37 year old

MEN ON SEX

described how children could reduce the opportunities for sex: 'There are definitely some situations with young kids when you're *both* keyed up, and you know what would be good for you at that time of day. But it just ain't going to happen – because you've got your kids in the garden playing football, their mates coming round. You think – stuff it, I'm going to the pub.'

A married 35 year old agreed that children did not always create circumstances conducive to sex: 'It's pressures of children being around and not having enough time on your own. Probably lots of men and women would like to be in a situation where they felt like having sex more often. In other words, I would like to have sex more often. I would like to be in a situation where it were feasible and possible.'

Some men did believe, though, that women's desire for sex diminished after they'd had children. In the words of a married 43 year old: 'A lot of women don't have the same drive for sex once they feel they've had enough children. They might still enjoy sex, but not quite as often.'

Young men are much more likely to say their sex life went downhill after their first child was born: 48 per cent of men under 24 make this complaint, in contrast with 32 per cent of men over 40. Indeed, 49 per cent of the over 40s say the new baby made little difference to their sexual relationship. A combination of factors come into play in this situation. The new mother may devote more attention to the baby than her partner, lose interest in sex, or it could be that both partners are too tired for sex. However, it seems that young men are less prepared than older men to accept this change of circumstances.

The men among the most likely to say their sex life stayed the same are those earning the least and men working in manual or clerical jobs. However, half the two-timing men found that sex does not improve after children.

The birth of a first child can have a disastrous effect on cohabitors' sex lives: 73 per cent of these men say the quality of their sex life took a turn for the worse afterwards. Only 33 per cent of married men say this is the case. As demonstrated in Chapter 4, men living with their partners but without children are well represented in the group having sex at least four times a week. Live-in Lovers clearly don't take kindly to having their sex life disrupted by the arrival of children!

The level of sexual activity he has seems to make a significant impact on a man's satisfaction with his sex life after his first child is born. Deterioration is only a problem for 27 per cent of men who have sex at least four times a week. But within the group of men who have sex less than once a month, there are proportionally twice as many complaints.

MY SEX LIFE DETERIORATED AFTER MY FIRST CHILD WAS BORN	
LEVEL OF ACTIVITY	
At least four times a week	27%
Two to three times a week	29%
Once a week	40%
Once or twice a month	43%
Less than once a month	56%

FATHER FIGURE

Next we explore the lifestyle, habits, needs and desires of the fathers in our sample. Fathers' priorities are firmly centred on their partner, children and having their own home. They are generally less concerned than those without children with having a good social life or career, money, freedom, independence, leisure and hobbies. Given the importance of their partner, it is not surprising that fathers don't rate male or female friends very highly. They are just as keen on sex as the non fathers, but more fathers are very confident that they know what their partner wants in bed.

Interestingly, only 58 per cent of fathers think women look for intelligence in a man, compared with 68 per cent of non fathers. They also give themselves a lower brainpower rating than men without children. Fathers are less likely than those without children to think women's main criteria are for a man to be handsome, self confident, romantic, athletic, artistic, shy or strong-willed. However, in their experience, it pays for a man to be in control. They also rate being strong and ambitious as less important than men without children, and rate themselves less ambitious.

The responsibilities of fatherhood must weigh heavily, as only half these men consider themselves fun-loving, compared with 70 per cent of men without children. However, they do believe this is a quality women look for in men. Only half may think they're the life and soul, but fathers do rate themselves as slightly more highly sexed than men without children. This could be because they feel women are less interested in sex after childbirth – an opinion expressed by some men in the discussion groups.

Compared with men without children, fathers see themselves as less caring, sensitive, handsome and romantic. When you have to look after children, provide for them and then take them out to the zoo occasionally, presumably there's less energy left for romantic dinners for two.

Men who have very young children are generally more likely to think women want a man who's responsible and in control rather than macho or strong. In their experience, women are not interested in a man being athletic, but they do want an understanding man. This group rate themselves as intelligent and responsible, but less fun-loving and romantic. Having young children is possibly linked to a lack of inhibition: only 9 per cent say they're shy, compared with 24 per cent of the whole sample.

Do women want affection in bed? Fathers and non fathers are united on this question: 72 per cent of both groups say this is important. However, fathers rate passion, stamina and energy as much less important than non fathers.

When it comes to what makes a woman sexually appealing, fathers tend to be lukewarm with regard to a woman's charm, dress sense, eyes and hair. Humour and intelligence are also less sexy for them than for men without children. In bed, fathers are more likely to prefer their partner to be naked and active, rather than passive. The features most likely to make fathers sit up and take notice are a good figure and a pretty face. Men with very young children rate charm and mouths as less important, but they also like to watch legs go by.

Fathers have less time for fantasy than men without children. This is presumably because these men are likely to have a regular partner and not much free time on their hands. They are less prone to think about sex at a pub, party or in bed, but are more likely to fantasise during sex with their partner.

Men with very young children are the least likely of all fathers to have any fantasies at all. But 36 per cent of these men do find time to daydream while travelling to work, and 43 per cent find their thoughts drifting towards sex when they're in the bath. Maybe these are the only moments they have to themselves!

Overall, these results suggest that becoming a father doesn't have to turn a man's life upside down, but it is likely to change his priorities and agenda. Faced with the dilemma of who is going to look after the baby, men accept they don't take enough responsibility for child care, but many still take refuge in work. As for sex after children, it comes down to the old quip: 'Have you got the time?' 'Yes – if you've got the energy!'

FIRST RESPONSE PROFILE

Name:	Jack
Age:	37
Occupation:	Training Consultant
Children:	One son, aged 12 months
Lives:	South East
Education:	'O', 'A' levels
Sexuality:	Heterosexual
Relationship:	Regular relationship, not cohabiting
Virginity loss:	21, average enjoyment
Comments:	30+ sexual partners; has sex less than once a month; strongly agrees he'd use a condom with new partner but rarely carries condoms around; tends to agree men don't do enough to look after their children

How's Your Fatherhood?

The findings seemed to relate to me and my experiences and, in general, seemed to show what I expected – older men and certain types of men would think women should be looking after the children. I don't agree with that. I think we should share childcare and I seem to be spot-on as 'Mr Average'.

I'm not married. I'm an active parent – separated from my partner – but still very 'friendly' with her! We share childcare – she does 70 per cent and I do 30 per cent. She wouldn't want me to have him any more because she has a very strong bond with him – she'd miss him too much. Sometimes I ask for him at weekends and she says: 'I didn't have him to be with someone else, I had him to be with me.' But that doesn't create a conflict because I do get to see him a lot, and I think the amount of childcare I do is all right for me.

I wouldn't want to be a sole carer, it would be too much for me and I'd get bored. I think I'd need more stimulation. I like independence, like to be on my own, need my own space. I'm pursuing a business and it would get in the way. But having said that, the responsibilities I do have, I take very seriously. If anything happened to my girlfriend, I *would* be sole carer and I would accept that. And my feeling is that when he's older I'll have him more. When a child is very young there is a very strong bond between mother and child, and my bond with him isn't as strong, but I think that may change when verbal communication starts to happen.

Odd Man Out

My friends are mostly single. I have one friend who works in the City, seven till seven; he's the only close friend I have who has children. He lives in Basingstoke and his wife is a housewife, and he doesn't do anything with the kids because when he comes home they're in bed. It's a very traditional relationship. If I were in the same situation I'd hate it. I wouldn't be in a relationship in the first place with a woman who'd accept being a housewife for 10-15 years, I'd find that boring.

Are You a New Man?

I hate the term 'New Man', but possibly I am one. New Men to me don't seem to be very strong. It conjures up women being in charge and being too alternative. But then, I do like some things about New Men – the good things. They look after their children, are open to crying, talking about their feelings, believe in equal partnerships and relationships. In relation to children, it means listening and talking to them, treating them with respect and as human beings, giving them quality time, being involved in the day-to-day care, being openly loving to them and *telling* them that you love them. I think that's very important.

The Generation Gap

My mother was the primary carer and my father didn't do the practical nappy-changing, feeding stuff that I do. Also my dad never talked about his feelings – he was a workaholic. I really would have liked him to have taken more interest, though he was a good father and was loving, kind and gentle; and I think I've got those traits from him. But living in that generation, men were brought up very traditionally. Go out to work and come back, while the wife looks after the children. That's how it was with my parents.

What's the Attraction?

I found it odd that the fathers in the survey reckoned that women wanted men to be in control. I don't think like that myself, I think both should try to strive towards equality. Generally I think women look for men who are 6 foot tall, and still look for the stereotypical successful man who has a lot of money and is prepared to look after them – the traditional type. But, increasingly, I think women are looking for men who are emotionally mature – this is what I would *like* to think. I mix with a fairly narrow band of people in a fairly narrow socio-economic group, so how people think across the board, I don't really know. I think women like handsome, attractive, strong men who are intelligent. I don't think many women like male bimbos. I don't think my perception of what women want has changed since having a child, but I think it will change with age – hopefully to men who are 5'8" or less. Being 5'8" myself, I like to look on the optimistic side.

I'm surprised that fathers in the survey, compared with the men without children, see themselves as less caring and less sensitive. As a father I feel *more* caring and sensitive now I've had a child than before I had a child. That's because I'm having to look after a very small human being who is very vulnerable, and that brings out my caring side (unless he really gets on my nerves!).

I would say most women want affection in bed. My kind of

affection is loving, warmth and nurturing. I find different parts of different women attractive. It couldn't be said about me that I'm a 'legs' man or a 'breast' man – those things aren't particularly important to me. I think the things more important to me now are the mental and emotional things, and the intelligence and sense of love, warmth and affection a woman offers. I think I find mothers more attractive than single women because having children matures people and emotional maturity is something I find attractive.

Is There Sex after Children?

Now there's not so much opportunity for sex – less time and energy. But I suppose I'm emphasising the point because I am living separately. If I was in a regular relationship, then the way people in your survey have answered would seem to make sense for me. To a certain extent I think men are understanding after children are born. But after things get very routine and family-orientated, and there isn't much sex any more, I imagine it's a dangerous period for men looking for affairs – when all the new experiences are absorbed and the first flush of excitement is over.

It can create problems for the future if people don't talk about how they feel, if both people don't work really hard on their relationship. Talking, listening, surprises, being supportive, those are the sorts of things you have to do.

The actual sex isn't different after children – not for me it wasn't! But it's now less urgent for my partner than previously. My partner very much wanted to have a baby and a lot of the sex seemed to be with that in mind. I didn't want a baby, I just wanted sex. So for her things have changed, but for me not. On the other hand, energy is more at a premium when you have children and often it's nice just to go to sleep rather than have sex.

Blood and Guts

I like to think of myself as quite elemental and I don't mind a bit of shit and vomit and blood now and then. For example, I don't mind making love to a woman if she's having her period, that doesn't bother me. The messy side of babies doesn't bother me at all. That's probably because I've done all these things quite a few times and to change a nappy for me is as natural as going for a shit or a wee myself. But there are the occasional monster shits that start in the nappy and go up to the nape of the neck – he normally does those when he's suffering from diarrhoea – I do find that difficult, but those are quite rare. I can still cope even when the shit factor is ten plus, provided I'm not wearing my office clothes!

MEN ON SEX

14.

Down Your Way

Who's cheating on whom? Who *are* the biggest drinkers? Which men have the most sex? And which men masturbate the most often? Who's for foreplay? And who doesn't think size is important? Our survey shows that the answers to these questions vary significantly according to whether men live in the North, Midlands or South. But don't expect to have your prejudices confirmed. The real picture is not so simply explained, and may well present a few surprises.

LIFESTYLE LINE-UP

There are no regional differences in fitness or men's perception of their own weight. They smoke more marijuana in the South and eat more fast food in the North. Men in the Midlands are the least likely to have tried homoeopathy, while massage is most common in the South. Drinking every day is least common in the North, where men are more likely to drink a moderate two to three times a week. Drinking a low amount of alcohol (1-7 units a week) is most common in the Midlands.

TOP PRIORITY

Job satisfaction and having a job are least important for Southern men and most important in the North, while Midlanders are less worried about having a career. Northerners are the keenest of the three regions on having a good social life. Meanwhile, men in the Midlands come across as more domesticated creatures: they put a higher value than those in the North or South on their partner, owning their own home, their children and their parents. For Southerners, freedom is important.

Holidays abroad are of least interest to men in the North. Men throughout Britain rate male companions as equally important, but good female companions are least important to those in the Midlands. There is also little regional variation on the importance men place on their appearance, although men in the South are slightly more concerned than other men with their clothes.

As far as hero worship is concerned, Richard Branson and Gary Lineker gain fewer votes from the Northern region, while Robin Williams gains more. Melvyn Bragg is equally unpopular across the regions: he gains just 1 per cent in all areas. Midland men are the least keen on Prince Charles, but they do like Ben Elton more than those elsewhere. Southern men are less keen on action men like Nigel Mansell and Arnold Schwarzenegger.

WHO'S STRAIGHT, WHO'S CHEATING?

In our sample, Northern men are the least likely of the three regions to be cohabiting with a partner outside marriage, and only 28 per cent of men in the Midlands are single, compared with 40 per cent of Northern men.

According to our survey, 6 per cent of men in the North say they have a regular partner in addition to their wife or live-in partner. This compares to just 1 per cent of men living in the South and Midlands.

It's worth noting some slight differences in sexual orientation. 96 per cent of men in the Midlands say they are only interested in sex with women, compared with 94 per cent of men in the rest of the country. Two per cent of Southern men claim only to be interested in sex with men, while 3 per cent of men in the North say they're mainly interested in sex with women, but also somewhat interested in men.

Men in the Midlands are the most likely to say they're fairly highly sexed and the least likely to say they're very highly sexed.

MEN ON SEX

THE FIRST BITE

Northern men get there first, as this table shows.

MEN WHO LOST THEIR VIRGINITY AGED 14-15	
In the North	22%
In the Midlands	17%
In the South	12%

According to our survey, men in the Midlands are slightly more likely to have lost their virginity aged 16-17, while just over a quarter of Southerners left it a little later and had their first experience of sex between the ages of 18 and 19.

The majority of men in all regions lost their virginity with someone they knew well. A slightly higher percentage of men in the North say they didn't use contraception, and more Midlanders first had sex on a one-night stand. Southerners come across as the most organised: 24 per cent of these men planned the occasion, compared with just 18 per cent of those in the North and Midlands. Six of the eight men who lost their virginity to a prostitute are from the South. More of the men in the North took advantage of their partner's parents being away. By contrast, more Southern men made the most of the absence of their own parents on the occasion when they lost their virginity.

As far as venue is concerned, the bedroom held an appeal for 52 per cent of Midlanders, and 62 per cent of Northerners. Eight per cent of Northern men lost their virginity outdoors in the country. Meanwhile, 8 per cent of Midlands men chose some other outdoor venue for the occasion.

HOW MANY PARTNERS?

Northern men are the most prone to memory loss when it concerns counting up how many sexual partners they've had: 10 per cent of them can't remember.

Overall, Midlanders have had fewer partners than those living in other parts of the country, and comparatively more have had between two and four sexual partners; only two of them have had between 15 and 29 partners. However, there are no regional differences when it comes to the most devoted sexual experimenters: exactly 7 per cent of men in all regions have had more than 30 partners.

Midlands men are also slightly more likely to have had only one partner during the last year. Again, 9 per cent of Northern men can't remember!

HOW OFTEN?

Northern men seem to have most sex: they are the men most likely to have sex two to three times a week. However, 7 per cent of non-virgins in the North don't have sex these days. But Northern men are the most likely to say they get enough sex, while men in the Midlands are the most keen to have more sex!

MEN WHO WANT TO HAVE SEX MORE OFTEN	
In the North	52%
In the Midlands	64%
In the South	59%

Men in the South are slightly more enthusiastic masturbators: 16 per cent of them masturbate more than three times a week, compared with 11 per cent of those in the North or Midlands. Northern men are more likely than Southerners to say they never masturbate: a quarter of Northerners say they never do so.

VARIATIONS ON A SEXUAL THEME

So much for sex and masturbation. But what tickles the fancy of men in the various regions? First of all, we explored the world of foreplay. Two in five men in every region have drunk alcohol as part of foreplay, and there are few variations according to whether they enjoy dressing up or tying up their partner. But in the case of using drugs as an additional stimulation, Southern men are the most in favour. Southern men account for seven of the eight men who've taken coke or crack, 31 of the 53 who've smoked marijuana, and six of the 11 who've used uppers. Those in the South also account for 10 of the 13 men who have used whips as a prelude to sex.

As far as sexual variations are concerned, Midlands men have definite views on a variety of sexual practices. They are greater exponents of oral sex and also have more experience than men in other regions of sex aids. They are, however, less likely than other men to have read porn magazines during the last year. Looking ahead to the future, they anticipate experiencing more oral sex, as well as more voyeurism, sex aids and porn videos (both soft- and hard-core varieties). However, they are the men slightly more keen *not* to experience oral or anal sex with a man, or anal sex with a woman. By contrast, it's men in the South who are slightly more likely to have been to a live sex show and to have had sex with a prostitute.

Tying in with the very small numbers who say they are homosexual (2 per cent), not many men in any region have had homosexual sex.

FANCY THAT

What makes someone particularly sexually attractive to men in different areas? Northerners are generally least interested in intelligent women, nor are they as attracted to breasts, bottoms or legs as men in other regions. But they are keen on their partners being naked. Men in the Midlands are more turned on by partners who take the initiative, and are partly clothed and active during sex. They are also more keen on a good body and a woman's dress sense. Legs and eyes are also particularly likely to attract the attention of men in the Midlands. For Southerners, charm, wit and hair are among the key attractions.

CLOSE YOUR EYES

Fantasising is slightly more common in the South. Men here are more likely to be found fantasising while travelling to work. They are also the group most likely to think about sex with someone they haven't slept with while lying in bed. Southern men are also particularly apt to fantasise about someone with them at the time, a friend or a work colleague.

When Midlands men do fantasise, it's unlikely to be during sex with their regular partner or while travelling to work. They are less likely to start having ideas about someone at work. They are not as keen on Gabriella Sabatini and Nastassia Kinski as men in other regions, but they do, however, seem more keen on Julie Christie.

A quarter of Northern men sometimes think about someone else when they're having sex with their regular partner. And they're more likely to be thinking of Patsy Kensit or Gabriella Sabatini than Felicity Kendal.

WHAT DO WOMEN WANT?

Midland men are less convinced than those in the North or South that women want strong men. In their experience, women want intelligent, caring, romantic and responsible men. They also rate themselves as particularly caring, intelligent and understanding – but are less romantic than men in other regions. Midlands men also believe that women want tenderness rather than dominance, and a man who treats women as equals. They rate sensuality more highly than men in other regions, but are the least persuaded that women want stamina in bed.

Men in the South are less likely than those elsewhere to think women are particularly interested in passion or affection in bed: they are more convinced, though, that women appreciate stamina. They are more likely than Midlanders or Northerners to say that artistic men and those who are in control appeal to women. They are also more likely to believe women want ambitious men, and rate themselves as more ambitious than men in other regions, but not as fun-loving.

Northern men, however, think women are interested in men who are passionate and dominant in bed, as well as athletic, money-orientated, fun-loving and handsome. Two-thirds of

MEN ON SEX

Northerners see themselves as fun-loving and responsible, but a much smaller percentage think they're artistic.

Midlands men are less likely to claim they're well-endowed or that size matters. Southerners, by contrast, are the most likely to say that size *is* important. They are the most confident they can tell their partners what they want during sex, while Northern men are more sure they know what their partner wants. Northerners are the most reluctant to say their performance is worse than other men's, and only 1 per cent of them say their own satisfaction is more important than their partner's. Men in the South are the most likely to say both people's satisfaction is important. Around three-quarters of men in all regions acquired their sexual technique from sexual partners, although men in the Midlands are particularly likely to have learned about sex this way. Sexual technique is gleaned more from sex manuals and text books in the South, whereas Northerners say they learned from conversations with male friends, television, films and videos.

MEN AT PLAY

The condom is most popular in the South, where 46 per cent of men use it as a form of contraception or protection. By contrast, 21 per cent of Northerners use no contraception at all! Men in the Midlands are the least likely to carry condoms: 83 per cent say they never carry them with them, although it's men in the North who are least likely to keep condoms at home. Men in the Midlands may be more conscious of the AIDS risk factor: 74 per cent say they wouldn't have sex with a new partner without using a condom. However, men in the South are slightly less likely to be put off by a woman carrying condoms or one who is prepared to have sex on a first date.

MEN AT WORK

Men in the Midlands are the most likely of the three regions to be sexually attracted to women at work, but more than half of men throughout Britain agree they have female colleagues whom they regard as friends. Southern men are more likely to disagree strongly that there is any sexual harassment where they work. A quarter of Southerners also say there are definitely equal opportunities for men and women in their workplace.

Northerners come across as slightly more chauvinistic in attitude: they're more likely to prefer to have a male bus driver, train driver, MP or doctor. They also tend to find the idea of having a female best friend very odd. Northern men are more likely to agree that men don't do enough to look after their children, but 44 per cent support the idea of women with young children going out to work. Southerners are the most likely to think women with pre-school-age children should stay at home. In the Midlands, men are more likely to disagree that women now have a better chance of getting on in their careers than men, and one in five are strongly opposed to positive discrimination in favour of women. A quarter of Midlanders say they sometimes find it difficult to express their views in female company for fear of being accused of sexism. They're more likely to prefer a male lawyer or boss, and half disagree that men want less sex in advertising.

Men from all over Britain feel most masculine during physical exercise, but Midlanders are the least likely to feel masculine behind the wheel or at work. Northerners feel more manly in bed than Southerners, and when they're in a pub or out socialising with a partner.

Finally, here's a table to summarise some of the findings in this chapter.

	NORTHERN MAN	MIDLANDS MAN	SOUTHERN MAN
Rates important:			
Social life	40%	30%	32%
His partner	45%	50%	44%
His home	44%	50%	38%

MEN ON SEX

	NORTHERN MAN	MIDLANDS MAN	SOUTHERN MAN
Likes:			
His partner to take the initiative	33%	40%	32%
An active partner	75%	80%	76%
Fantasises:			
Sometimes, during sex with regular partner	25%	14%	24%
In bed	68%	64%	72%
Thinks he's:			
Highly sexed	23%	24%	25%
Fun-loving	67%	64%	56%
Intelligent	64%	71%	70%

Index

Note: figures in italics refer to tables

abuse victims 67, 87-93; age of abuse 88; kind of abuse 88; frequency of abuse *88*; partners and *92*; priorities of *90*, 91; who abused 89, *89*
activity *see* frequency
acupuncture 19, 69
advertising, sex and 9-10, 173
affection and tenderness 102, 103, 104
age xi; frequency and 37; idea of women changes 58-9, *57*; at marriage *xii*; virginity and xiii, 23-4, *23*
AIDS: be prepared 129-30; condoms and 134, 136, 137-8, 139, 172; first-date sex and 132; heterosexuals and 127, 129; risk factors 126-7; threat of 123-6
alcohol: as a warm-up 43-4, 54, 82, 85; regional differences 169; sexually abused and 90; virginity loss 25, 26, 28, 75
Alcorn, Keith 128
Alexander Technique 19
anal sex: disapproval of 53; fantasies of 52; with men 50-1; with women 45, 48, 50, 76, 77
aphrodisiacs 43, 45, 68
appearance; ideal women 56-7, *56*, importance of 12, 15; weight xii, 18, 62
aromatherapy 19
artistic men 76, 97
athletes, sexual 67-70, 97, 135-6
aversion to practices 53

bath, fantasising in 117-18, 119, 120
bed, fantasising in 117-18, *119*
bisexuality 49
blue movies 43, 44, 76, 113
Bly, Robert *Iron John* 10
body, equipped for sex 100-2
bondage 45, 46, 49, 50, 52, 75; as foreplay 43, 44; interested types 72; regional differences 170
Bragg, Melvyn 20, 167
Branson, Richard 20-1, 69, 83, 167

career 12, 68, 77, 85; *see also* employment; working place
cars 12, 14; *see also* driving
celibacy 17, 35, 39, 82, 124
Charles, Prince of Wales 20, 21, 83, 84, 167
charm, in women 60-1
chauvinism 1, 4, 71, 173
children: absent fathers and 156-7, *156*; cause decline in sex 34, 35, 157-9, *159*, 164; fathers and 159-60, 161-4; importance of 12, 16; women's rights over 5; working mothers and 154-6, *154*; *see also* fatherhood
Choong, Da 127
Christie, Julie 69, 122, 171
clothes 17; women's sense of 57
cohabitation xii, 6; *see also* live-in lovers
coil 134
Collins, Joan 84, 122
Comfort, Alex, *The Joy of Sex* 40
communication: about performance 105-7; about partner's wants 107-8; during sex 108; about satisfaction 109-10
condoms: AIDS and 123-6, *124*, *125*, 136, 137-8, 139, 172; as contraception 134-5; etiquette of 137-8; who carries 74, 77, 129-30, 138; women carry 130-1, 138
confidence 108
contraception 134-6; virgins and 25-6
control: crisis of self-belief 80; initiative in sex 63-4, *63*
Cosmopolitan (magazine) 40
Costelloe, Paul 4, 17

Davies, Sharron 100, 122
diaphragm 134
disapproval of practices *53*, 81
divorce and separation xi, 5, 9
DIY, masculinity of 3, 77
doctors, female 7, 8
dominance 102, 103
double standard 114
drinking *see* alcohol
driving: fantasising and 118;

175

MEN ON SEX

masculinity of 3-4, 77, 84; women and 7, 8
drugs 18-19; as foreplay 43, 44-5; marijuana 44-5, 68, 76, 77; regional differences 170; sexually abused and 90; spread of HIV 126, 127; virginity loss and 25; *see also* alcohol
Durex survey 125-6, *125*, 134

early-learners 67, 74-7
education and information about sex xi, 40
Elton, Ben 20, 21, 167
emotions 5
employment x, xi, 12, 98; job satisfaction 13; masculinity and 3; security of 15; unemployment 5-6; women and roles 7-8, *7*; *see also* work place
equality 99
Esquire (magazine) 129
etiquette, condoms and 137-8
exercise xii
exes 67, 85-7
experience *xiii*, xi, 107; self-concept and 99-100

The Face (magazine) 129
fantasies *50*, 78, 86, 160; of the inactive 83-4; objects of 120-2; regional differences 171; two-timers and 72, 115; where and when? 116-20, *117*, *119*
fathers xi, xiii, 3, 154-6, *154*; absence 156-7, *156*; children cause decline in sex 157-9, *159*, 164; ideal woman 160; power struggle and 6; regional differences 173; role of 159-60, 161-4; virginity and contraception 26
feminism 1, 6, 77
Fenn, Sherilyn 121
fidelity and infidelity xii, 79-82; novelty 113-15; regional differences 167
films, blue 43, 76; learning from 113
first-date sex 131-3, *132*, *133*, 139
food 68-9
foreplay and warm-up 43-4, *43*; regional differences 169-70
freedom 12, 13
frequency xiii, 34-5, *34*, *98*; age and 37; belief in women's desires 99-100; male-female differences 36-7; masturbation and 42; not more partners 32; overload 36; pornography and 47-8; regional differences 169, *169*; satisfaction with 35-6; within a relationship 39; *see also* partners
friendship: importance of 12, 16; with female colleagues 146-7, *146*, 172; with women 8-9, *8*, 80-1
fun-loving 97

gardening, masculinity of 3, 77
Gibson, Mel 20, 21
group sex *see* troilism

Hanson, Lord 20, 21, 71
health 12, 14, 82
Henry, Lenny 20, 21
heroes 20-2
holidays 12, 16; virginity loss and 25, 27
home 12, 13
homeopathy 19
homosexuality xiii, 45, 49-50; AIDS and 126-7, 128-9, 137; fantasies of 52-3; live-in lovers 77; regional differences 170; and sexual abuse 91
humour, in women 57, 58, 59, 60, 83

i-D (magazine) 129, 137
impotence 106
income *see* employment; money
independence 12, 13
infidelity *see* fidelity and infidelity
intelligence, in women 57, 58, *59*, 60, 83
Iron John (Bly) 10

Jagger, Mick 20, 21, 83
job satisfaction 82, 85
jobs *see* employment
The Joy of Sex (Comfort) 40

Kendal, Felicity 72, 122, 171
Kensit, Patsy 121, 122, 171
Kinski, Nastassia 72, 84, 122, 171

Lane, Lord 49

lawyers, female 8
leisure and hobbies 12, 14
Lineker, Gary 20, 21, 83, 167
live shows 48, 50; disapproval 53; fantasies of 52; regional differences 170
live-in lovers 67, 77-9
Livingstone, Ken 141-2
Lone Rangers 67, 82-4
love, virginity loss and 25, 26, 28

machismo 97
making love v sex 103, 110-12
Mansell, Nigel 20, 21, 71, 167
Marks, Alfred 145, 148
marriage xi, *xii*, 26
marriage counselling 19, 85
masculinity 77, 84; regional differences 173; situations 1-4, *2*; threats to 37
massage 19, 69
masturbation 54, 83, 93; fantasy and 117-18, 120; frequency 41-2, *41*; regional differences 169; sexual athletes and 69
Members of Parliament, women as 7, 142
Midlands men *see* regional differences
money x, 6, 8, 81; importance of 12, 14; women's 58, 60, 61
monogamy 31, *31*, 38
MORI poll, sample questioned ix-xi
Murdoch, Rupert 20

New Men 1, 9, 10, 80; children and 154, 162-3
Northern men *see* regional differences
novelty v fidelity 113-15
NSPCC (Nat'l Society for the Prevention of Cruelty to Children) 87, 89

onanism *see* masturbation
one-woman man 79-82
oral sex: disapproval of 53; fantasies of 52; regional differences 170; with men 49; with women 45, 46, 47, 50, 76, 81
orgasms, women's 108

parents 25, 26; as abusers 89; father's influence on men 10-11, *10*; importance of 16-17
parties 25, 26; fantasising at 118
partners 4, 12, 13, 99; determine kind of sex 103; fantasising during sex 118, 119; learning from 73, 113, 172; number of xi, 30-3, *30*, *33*, 38, 39, 86, *92*; regional differences 168-9; self-concept and 99
passion 102, 103
Paxman, Jeremy 20, 21-2, 79
peace and quiet 12, 16, 91
penis size 73, 100-2
performance, communication about 105-7
The Pill 134, 136, 138, 139
Pitt-Kethley, Fiona 100, 105
politicians 7, 22 142
politics 17; racism and sexism in 142
pornography 45, 46, 47, 50, 52; disapproval of 54; films 43, 44, 76, 113; for the inactive 84; interested types 68, 72; regional differences 170
Porritt, Jonathan 20, 22
positive discrimination 4, 69, 81, 141-3, *141*, 152; regional differences 173
power 17; between the sexes 4-8, *4*
priorities *12*; in bed 102-4; regional differences 166-7; sexually abused and *90*, 91
prostitutes 45, 46, 49, 68, 76; disapproval of 53; fantasies of 50, 51, 52; regional differences 170; virginity loss and 25
psychoanalysis and therapy 19, 22, 75, 85
pubs: fantasising at 11; masculinity of 3, 4, 77, 84

quickies 110-12

radio 113
Rayner, Claire 94, 117, 132, 139
regional differences: condoms & AIDS 172; fantasies 171; fidelity 167; foreplay and activities 169-70; frequency of sex 169, *169*; ideas on women's wants 171-2; lifestyle and priorities 166-7; partners 168-7;

priorities *174*; virginity loss and 168, *168*
relationships, determine sex 103; *see also* partners
religion 17-18, 75, 83
responsibility 96
rewards 111
Roberts, Julia 79, 121, 122
romance 97

Sabatini, Gabriella 72, 122, 171
sado-masochism 44, 45, 72, 77; banned 49; disapproval of 53; fantasies of 50, 51, 52
Salako, John 2-3
satisfaction 109-10
Schwarzenegger, Arnold 20, 21, 167
Scruton, Roger, *Sexual Desire* 55, 57
The Secret Garden 40
self-assessment *96*
self-confidence 97
Selleck, Tom 100
sensitivity 98
sensuality 102, 103
separation *see* divorce and separation
sex, importance of *12*, 15
sex aids 45, 48, 50, 51, 77; disapproval of 53; regional differences 170
sex education 113
sexism 6
Sexual Desire (Scruton) 55, 57
sexual harassment 144-6, *144*, 151, 172
smoking xii, 18, 68, 85
social life 12, 14
Southern men *see* regional differences
sport 22; masculine activity 2-3, 4, 77; not a sex substitute 18
stamina and energy 102, 103, 104
submission 102
Sugar, Alan 20, 21, 71

Taylor, Sir Teddy 142
techniques 172; learning 112-13
telephone, fantasising and 118
television 113, 118
Terrence Higgins Trust 127
Thatcher, Margaret 122
therapy 19-20
troilism 48-9, 76, 77, 80; disapproval of 53; fantasies of 50, 51
two-timers 6, 67, 71-4; partners and 32, 33; *see also* fidelity and infidelity

vasectomies 134
videos 113
virginity loss xiii; age of xi, 23-4, *24*; circumstances 25-9, *25*; early learners and 74-5; enjoyment of xi, 27, 52; later number of partners 31, 32; location of 27-8, *27*; regional differences 168, *168*; religion and 17-18
voyeurism 45, 46, 48, 68, 77; disapproval of 53; fantasies of 50, 51; regional differences 170

Walters, Julie 4
Wax, Ruby 122
Wentz, Siggy 100
whips, as foreplay 43, 44; regional differences 170
Williams, Robin 20, 21, 167
women: active v passive 64-6, *65*, 78; balance of power 4-8, *4*; bosses 143-4, *143*, 152-3; career progression *141*; carry condoms 130-1, 138; changing needs 94; expectations of sex 102-4; fantasising at 118, 119; frequency and desire 36-7; friendship with 8-9, *8*; ideal 56-62, *56*, 69, 73, 80, 160; initiative in sex 63-4, *63*, 78, 85; job roles 7-8, *7*, 79, 142; nakedness 62-3, *62*, 73; orgasms 108; what do they want? 95-100, *95*, 171-2; working mothers 69, 80, 81, 154-6, *154*, 173; *see also* positive discrimination; work place: fantasising at 118, 119; female bosses 143-4, *143*, 152-3; hours 140-1, *140*; male-female friendship 146-7, *146*; regional differences 172-3; sexual attraction 147-50, *147*; sexual harassment 144-6, *144*, 151, 172; sexual relations 152; women's progress 141-3; *141; see also* employment; positive discrimination

yoga 19, 83

zero population growth 133